1,001

HOME HEALTH REMEDIES
for SENIORS

By the Editors of FC&A Medical Publishing

Publisher's Note

This book is for information only. It does not constitute medical advice and should not be construed as such. We cannot guarantee the safety or effectiveness of any drug, treatment, or advice mentioned. Some of these tips may not be effective for everyone.

A good doctor is the best judge of what medical treatment may be needed for certain conditions and diseases. We recommend in all cases that you contact your personal doctor or health care provider before taking or discontinuing any medications, or before treating yourself in any way.

Jesus was going through all the cities and villages, teaching in their synagogues and proclaiming the gospel of the kingdom, and healing every kind of disease and every kind of sickness.

Matthew 9:35

FC&A Medical Publishing
103 Clover Green
Peachtree City, GA 30269

Produced by the staff of FC&A

Cover Images: © 1996 RubberBall Productions

Third Printing April 2001

ISBN 1-890957-45-3

Table of contents

Introduction

People are living longer than ever. The baby boomers are moving into their golden years, and they are staying healthy through knowledge — the kind of knowledge you're holding in your hands right now.

Because we care about you, our valued customer, we want you to have the latest information on how to stay healthy for many years to come. That's why we wrote *1,001 Home Health Remedies for Seniors*.

Everything you need for total health care — from your head to your feet — can be found in these pages. The chapters are conveniently organized alphabetically by condition. You can flip right to your area of concern, or you can read the book from cover to cover. You're sure to find useful information for yourself and your family.

This valuable book was written with seniors in mind, but it contains something for everyone. We hope you enjoy the "fruits of our labor."

The Editors of FC&A

Allergies

Take charge of annoying allergy symptoms

If itchy eyes, a runny nose, sneezing, and coughing are part of your everyday life, you could be super sensitive to common substances, like plant pollen, dust mites, mold, animal dander, feathers, or chemicals. Normally harmless to most people, these allergens can cause the mucous membranes in your eyes, nose, throat, and sinuses to go wild.

Although there is no cure for allergies, you can control them by avoiding the things that trigger your symptoms in the first place.

- Choose nonaerosol household cleaning products.

- Avoid cigarette or cigar smoke.

- Keep the humidity inside your house at less than 50 percent to reduce mold.

- Stay away from birds, cats, and dogs.

- Try to plan your outdoor activities away from seasonal grasses and weeds that release pollen.

- After working in your yard or garden, remove your clothes, shower, and rinse your nostrils with salt water.

- Install a filter system on your air conditioner.

- Dust with a wet cloth to trap allergens. A dry cloth simply spreads the dust around into the air.

- Replace wall-to-wall carpeting with wood or vinyl floors. Put down area rugs that can be cleaned or washed regularly.

• Repair leaking faucets or pipes to reduce the growth of mold.

And here's another thing you should consider — dust mites. These tiny insects live in bedding, rugs, carpets, cushions, stuffed toys, and mattresses. They eat dead, sloughed-off human skin cells and give off waste material that can trigger allergic reactions.

The good news is mites can be killed by hot-water washing or dry cleaning. This means fabric items more frequently washed or dry-cleaned are less likely to contain dust mites and other allergens. Wool clothing and linens, for instance, usually contain more mites because they are washed less often. Remember though, if you wash your bedding in cold water, you may remove most of the mite waste materials but not the live mites.

Here's how to kill dust mites and remove their allergens:

• Choose clothes and linens that can be washed regularly in very hot water.

• Store out-of-season clothes and linens under dry conditions, since mites need moisture.

• Wash or dry clean items after they've been stored for a season.

• Tumble items in a hot dryer.

• Cover your mattress and pillows with plastic.

• Place items in a deep freeze for at least 24 hours.

• •
Beware of this deadly allergy

What's the difference between a peanut and a soybean? Not much if you're allergic. In some people, both of these legumes can cause a severe allergic reaction called anaphylaxis, causing difficulty breathing, swelling, rash, rapid heartbeat, convulsions, and even death.

While thousands know they are allergic to peanuts, few people know they could also react to soybeans. Children who are allergic to peanuts, especially those with asthma, are most at risk, according to a Swedish study.

It's not always easy to know if a processed food contains soy. Some ground and processed meats, like hamburgers, sausages, and meatballs, use soy as a filler. It can show up in everything from cheese to toothpaste to veggie burgers.

Even though food labels are not always accurate, read them carefully. If you're not sure if the product contains soy, don't take a chance.

● ●

14 ways to breathe cleaner air at home

If you have trouble concentrating or suffer from coughing, sneezing, headaches, nausea, itchy eyes, or a stuffy nose, you may be allergic to your home. This condition, called sick building syndrome, can also lead to asthma, heart disease, and cancer.

Today's energy-efficient buildings allow less outdoor air to flow in and more pollutants to build up inside. Recent studies have found that the air inside many homes and offices is more polluted than the outdoors, even in the most polluted cities.

Although you won't always be able to smell indoor air pollutants, a quick and easy way to tell if your home has poor ventilation is to step outside for a few minutes. If you notice any odors when you come back in, your home needs better ventilation.

If you think your home has a serious pollution problem, contact your state or local health department to have it tested. In the meantime, try some of these easy, do-it-yourself remedies. You'll be increasing air movement and cleaning the air, which could help you feel better.

Fix your fireplace. Never burn pressure-treated wood in your fireplace — it contains chemicals. Clean and maintain your chimney and flue and repair any cracks.

Keep it clean. Clean your house regularly. Use a central vacuum system that is vented outdoors or has a high-efficiency filter.

Pass on the pesticides. Don't use more of a pesticide than recommended. You won't be killing more pests — you'll just be increasing the level of chemicals you and your family will be exposed to. Use natural means of pest control when possible.

Cut down on moisture. Standing water, water-damaged materials, or wet surfaces are perfect breeding grounds for mold, mildew, bacteria, and insects. One of the worst allergens, house dust mites, just love damp, warm environments. You can control the growth of these irritants by controlling the humidity in your home. To do this, empty and clean the evaporation/condensation trays in air conditioners and refrigerators often. Clean humidifiers regularly and change the water daily. If your carpets get flooded, clean and dry them as quickly and thoroughly as possible, or replace them. Make sure your basement is clean and dry.

Store chemicals safely. Follow label instructions for using and storing paints, cleansers, and other chemicals. Make sure lids are on tightly and dispose of old containers properly. Check your home for asbestos and lead-based paint.

Choose real wood. Pressed wood products, like particleboard, plywood paneling, and fiberboard, emit formaldehyde.

Change your filters. Clean or change the air filters on your heating and air conditioning units every few months — more often if you find them dirty. Have your units serviced regularly to keep them running smoothly.

Give your gas stove a tune-up. If you have a gas stove, make sure it is adjusted properly to reduce emissions. The flame tip should be blue, not yellow. A yellow tip means more pollutants. Call your gas company if you need your burner adjusted. If you're in the market for a new stove, buy one with a pilotless ignition. This means there is no continuously burning pilot light. And remember, don't ever use a gas stove to heat your home.

Install UV bulbs. Canadian researchers tested ultraviolet lights, which they say can kill germs, inside central heating, ventilation, and air conditioning systems. After only three weeks, there were less bacteria and fungi on the surfaces of the ventilation system. Workers had fewer headaches and eye irritations and less difficulty concentrating. This is safe, costs very little, and no one knows they're there. Talk to an electrician about installing ultraviolet lights in your home's ventilation system.

Let in some fresh air. Unless you're extremely allergic, open up the windows and doors occasionally to blow out stale air and irritants. Provide good ventilation when you're doing things that increase pollution, like painting, stripping, sanding, or cleaning.

Pick a dry cleaner carefully. Don't use a dry cleaner that returns your clothes with a strong chemical smell. They either aren't drying the items properly or aren't removing as much of the cleaning solvent as they should. Hang freshly dry cleaned clothes in the garage or outdoors for a day or so.

Clean the air. Air cleaners vary from small portable models to whole-house systems. The best ones collect lots of pollutants and have a high air circulation rate. How well they work will depend on how strong the pollution is in your home and how well the systems are maintained.

Vent to the outside. Turn on bathroom and kitchen exhaust fans, but make sure they vent to the outdoors, not back into your home. Vent your clothes dryer to the outside. Run a window air conditioning unit with the vent open. Install window, attic, and crawl space fans. Vent a room by slightly opening a door or window where you're running a gas or kerosene space heater.

Boost circulation. Look into installing a mechanical system that brings outdoor air into your home. Some include energy-efficient heat recovery ventilators, also known as air-to-air heat exchangers. For more information, contact the Conservation and Renewable Energy Inquiry and Referral Service (CAREIRS), P.O. Box 3048, Merrifield, VA 22116. Their toll-free number is 800-523-2929.

• •
Put the brakes on sick car syndrome

Have you ever turned on your car's air conditioner and been blasted with a smelly socks odor that had you frantically rolling down the windows? Not what you'd expect — especially from a new car. But it's mostly new cars that suffer from this phenomenon called sick car syndrome.

Similar to sick building syndrome, the awful smell is caused by fungi and bacteria growing on your car's air conditioning coils. If that's not bad enough, it can also cause headaches, nausea, asthma attacks, and allergy symptoms.

Some cars get it and some cars don't. The only thing you can do is use the AC setting that brings in air from the outside. This helps recirculate the contaminated air. Then run the blower without the air conditioner on to dry the moisture off the coils.

• •

Amazing way to reduce indoor pollution

Plants add beauty to a home. They also do a great job cleaning and purifying the air. Even NASA believes in the benefits of houseplants. They discovered that if they put plants inside a closed environment, the leaves removed "low levels" of pollution, and the roots removed even more, especially if activated carbon filters were placed around them.

In studies, it took about 15 to 20 houseplants to clean the air in an average-sized home — about 1,800 square feet. The only caution is don't overwater. Damp soil can promote mold and mildew, exactly the kind of thing you're trying to get rid of.

The four major chemicals plants remove from the atmosphere are carbon dioxide, benzene (found in gasoline, inks, oils, paints, plastics, rubber, dyes, detergents, and pharmaceuticals), formaldehyde (found in particleboard, plywood, foam insulation, grocery bags, room deodorizers, wax paper, facial tissues, paper towels, and permanent press fabrics), and trichloroethylene, also known as TCE, (found in dry cleaning chemicals, printing inks, paints, lacquers, varnishes and adhesives).

To get rid of toxins inside your home or office, choose from the following plants.

English ivy	Philodendron	Spider plant
Aloe vera	Shefflera	Potted mum
Dracaena	African daisy	Bamboo plant
Corn plant	Chrysanthemum	Snake plant
Date palm	Pothos	

• •

Taking a shower? Don't forget to open a window

Environmental engineers at The University of Texas have proven that showers, washing machines, bathtubs, and dishwashers release harmful chemicals from public water supplies into the air causing indoor pollution.

That's because tap water sometimes contains very small amounts of contaminants, like radon and by-products of chlorination. Researchers believe breathing in air-borne particles of the water expose you to more of these potentially dangerous chemicals than simply drinking the water.

Here's how you can protect yourself from this indoor pollution:

• When showering or running a bath, run an exhaust fan or open a window.

• Don't open your dishwasher immediately after running a cycle, and don't breathe in that puff of air when you open the door.

• Don't add chlorinated bleaches or detergents to dishwashers and washing machines.

• Turn on your stove's exhaust fan when you're boiling water.

• Don't run a less than fully loaded dishwasher because more water is air-borne.

It doesn't seem to matter how you adjust your shower spray or how hard you turn on the water. The amount of chemicals released into the air stays about the same.

• •

Secrets for surviving pet allergies

You love your pet, but your nose doesn't. Every time you walk in your house, the itchy, sneezy, stuffy misery begins. Here's how the two of you can learn to get along.

Pick flooring carefully. Get rid of all carpets, if possible. They trap up to 100 times more pet allergens than polished floors. If you must have carpets, choose those that:

- have a low pile density.

- are low in height (less than one-quarter inch tall).

- are coated with fluorocarbon (like Teflon).

- have thick carpet fibers.

These factors affect how easy it is to remove pet dander and hair. To help keep your home allergen-free, vacuum every few days and have your carpets professionally cleaned often. No matter how you cover it, avoid sitting or lying on the floor.

Get to the bottom of dust. Now that you've gotten rid of those carpets, how do you clean your bare floors? Researchers recommend using cleaning systems with disposable cloths that attract and trap dust electrostatically. When compared with cotton cloths, rubber- or nylon-bristled brooms, sponge brooms, oiled-cloth sweepers, dry synthetic mops, and synthetic wool sweepers, these cloths removed more cat and dog allergens.

Don't worry about your ducts. The advertising is convincing — clean your home ventilation system to reduce pet allergens. But when researchers tested several homes containing dogs or cats, they found the air duct filters did a good job of keeping pet allergens from blowing back through the house. The experts at the American Academy of Allergy, Asthma, and Immunology say don't spend a lot of time or money on cleaning your air ducts. It won't really reduce the amount of animal allergens in your home.

Pick a perfect pillow. Choosing a pillow is as personal and as hotly debated as topping the perfect hot dog — catsup only or loaded with the works? Synthetic or feather? But now your pillow purchase should take into account your pets. No — you don't have to share your pillow with Fluffy, but you don't want to share pet allergens, either. Researchers at the North West Lung Centre in England found that synthetic pillows collected six to eight times more dog and cat allergens than feather pillows. The difference might be in the feathers, or it could be the tightly woven covers on feather pillows. Whatever the reason, for sweet, sneeze-free dreams, pluck a plumper feather pillow.

Beware of exotic pets. It's not just cats and dogs that can tickle your nose and bring on the sneezes. Look to other animals, especially exotic pets, for the dander behind your allergies. One man suffered a near-fatal asthma attack while washing his ferret. Minks, gerbils, and Guinea pigs have also brought on allergic reactions.

Let baby make four. Contrary to popular belief, there is new evidence that living with an indoor pet for the first year of a baby's life will reduce his risk of developing allergies later on. The Medical College of Georgia followed almost 500 children until they were six years old. Only between 6 and 13 percent tested positive for pet allergens. This means many new parents won't have to choose between Fido and Junior.

● ●
Cat dander has more than nine lives

You can run, but you can't hide from cat dander — tiny particles of skin that trigger the irritating symptoms of cat allergy. Researchers have discovered that this allergen is difficult, if not impossible, to completely remove from the air, even after a cat has been gone for years.

Surprising numbers of people test positive for cat allergy even if they've never owned a cat. This means that simply being around a cat owner or visiting his home can produce a sensitivity that could lead to a full-blown allergic reaction. It's enough to make you ... paws.
● ●

Survival guide for unusual allergies

What do bugs, a luxurious fabric, shampoo, and your new best friend have in common? They can all trigger allergic reactions and asthma attacks. Allergens come in a variety of shapes and sizes, and they can show up in some pretty unexpected places.

Beware of the Asian ladybug. About 20 years ago, a new species of ladybug was imported from Asia into the southeastern United States to help control aphids on apple and pecan trees. But unlike the common American red ladybug, this orange-colored species lives year round and has been known to infest homes by the thousands. Some people have developed allergic reactions to the insect from breathing insect parts in the air. Experts believe the Asian ladybug could create a widespread problem if it continues to multiply and spread to other states.

So how do you get rid of these troublesome intruders? Don't use insecticides since dead ladybugs attract other pests, like carpet beetles. Instead, vacuum and dust often and caulk up cracks and crevices around your house, especially in the attic.

The Asian ladybug is not the only insect known to cause allergic reactions. Cockroaches, miller moths, and dust mites are all nonstinging, indoor pests that can bring on asthma-like symptoms.

Watch out for wild silk. Silk sheets, a silk tie, maybe even silk pajamas — nothing says comfort and elegance in quite the same way. And nothing says allergic reactions, either. If you own products made from wild silk, you should know they have not been pre-washed and heated like other kinds of silk. That means the material may still contain parts of the silkworm or insects that feed on silkworm cocoons and waste matter. These particles are known to trigger asthma attacks in some people.

Don't shy away from new friends. If you have a runny nose, red eyes, and you hate meeting new people, your problems may be caused by specific brain chemicals. Researchers from Harvard University believe that hay fever and shyness are both controlled by the same transmitters — those that regulate mood, smell, and immunity.

Think twice before you lather up. A trip to a spa or hair salon should leave you feeling refreshed and wonderful. Not so for some people who are allergic to products containing collagen, keratin, elastin, milk, wheat, almond, or silk. These ingredients, sometimes added to hair-care products, soaps, bath gels, and creams, can cause hives, swollen lips, wheezing, and other breathing difficulties in certain people.

And are you considering coloring your hair blonde? Do you cover your gray? If you use a hair dye product, you could develop an allergic reaction to it, even if you've been symptom free for years. This type of reaction is rare, but it can strike without warning and — in extreme cases — can be fatal.

The most common allergic ingredient in many permanent hair dyes is a synthetic organic compound called p-phenylenediamine. To protect yourself from this kind of potential disaster, do a patch test every time you color your hair, and follow all printed safety instructions exactly. Another option is to switch to a semi-permanent type of hair dye.

If you have any allergic symptoms, like swollen eyes, itchiness, hoarseness, heart palpitations, or shortness of breath, don't waste time. Your body's response to the allergen can be extremely rapid. Call for emergency help immediately.

Alzheimer's disease

Memory loss or Alzheimer's?
How to tell the difference

Every time you forget a name or lose your glasses, you may panic, thinking you have Alzheimer's. Chances are, you're perfectly fine. In fact, worrying about your memory loss is actually a good sign that you're OK.

The first stage of Alzheimer's is more than having small lapses in your memory. You experience regular memory problems, like constantly forgetting appointments or telling the same story over and over. At this stage, you're still able to function normally, solve problems, concentrate on tasks, and communicate — in short, your personality is still the same. As the disease progresses, not only do you lose your memory, but these other abilities, as well.

Detecting Alzheimer's early, before all the symptoms set in, is the best hope for the future. Once the disease is evident, too much damage has already been done to memory cells. Unfortunately, a recent study found that one out of five families with a member suffering from mental problems was unable to recognize the problem. Look at this list of early warning signs that you or a loved one may have the disease.

- **Forgetfulness.** While it's normal to forget names or lose your keys once in a while, frequent forgetfulness may be a red flag. Think of it this way — it's normal to forget your keys, but if you can't remember what the keys are for, it's time to get help.

- **Speech problems.** Sometimes a word is on the tip of your tongue, but you just can't get it out. Everyone has that experience occasionally, but if you often have trouble with simple words, or your speech isn't understandable, you may have a problem.

- **Misplacing things.** Some people lose track of their keys or the TV remote control almost every day. But finding lost items in a strange place, like the microwave or the refrigerator, should be cause for concern.

- **Personality changes.** Everyone goes through changes in their lives. Some people become more easygoing and relaxed as they age, while others seem to turn into grumpy old men and women. Alzheimer's can cause profound personality changes, transforming a calm, sweet person into someone who is frightened, paranoid, or confused.

- **Loss of judgment.** You may think young people show poor judgment in their choice of clothes, but if you can't judge what clothing is appropriate for you to wear, you may be the one with a problem. For example, if you put your socks on your hands, or wear shorts when it's snowing, you have lost your ability to judge.

- **Problems with familiar tasks.** Busy people are often distracted and may forget to finish something they started. Someone with Alzheimer's might prepare a meal and not only forget to serve it, but not remember she even made it in the first place. Or she may have problems remembering how to prepare the meal at all.

- **Mood swings.** Going from one extreme to the other rapidly, for no apparent reason, is cause for concern.

- **Disorientation.** If you become lost in a strange city, no one would accuse you of having Alzheimer's. But if you are lost in your own neighborhood, that's another story. Place or time disorientation is an early symptom of Alzheimer's. If you easily forget what day it is or how to get to a familiar place, see your doctor.

- **Loss of interest.** Anyone can lose interest in a slow-paced movie, but when you aren't interested in any of the things that used to bring you pleasure, that's a little more serious.

- **Trouble "adding it up."** If doing simple math problems suddenly becomes more difficult, you may have a problem yourself. Math requires abstract thinking, connecting symbols (numbers) with a meaning. Abstract thinking is one of the first skills you lose with Alzheimer's.

A new variation of the familiar MRI (magnetic resonance imaging) allows doctors to diagnose very early stages of Alzheimer's. This "functional MRI" can give a closer look at a specific area in the memory center of your brain. Experts believe a breakdown here is not caused by normal aging but is a sign of early Alzheimer's. So even if you show no outward symptoms of the disease, this test gives such advance warning that you can begin treatment before it's too late.

• •
Supplement shows great promise

If almost half of all Alzheimer's victims were lacking a particular body chemical, you might wonder if the two were somehow related. That's exactly the question scientists are asking about coenzyme Nicotinamide Adenine Dinucleotide (NADH).

NADH is produced by every living cell and is important in energy production — the more NADH a cell has, the more energy it can produce. As you age, your cells produce less and less NADH, but in people with Alzheimer's, this decline is even greater.

Although NADH supplements are still controversial, tests have shown that they can improve brain function and treat other symptoms of Alzheimer's disease without side effects. But there is a drawback — stopping NADH treatment caused the symptoms to return even worse than before.

Talk with your doctor about this supplement to see if it's right for you or someone you care about.

• •

8 surprising ways to avoid Alzheimer's

One out of every 10 people over the age of 65 has Alzheimer's disease. If you want to avoid becoming an Alzheimer's statistic, consider some of these promising and inexpensive ways to prevent or slow down this devastating disease.

Aspirin. If trying to remember your grocery list gives you a headache, you might reach for some aspirin. According to some studies, if you took aspirin every day, you might remember that list more easily. Some doctors think inflamed brain tissue contributes to Alzheimer's. They say a daily dose of aspirin or other nonsteroidal anti-inflammatory drug (NSAID), like ibuprofen, could help prevent or treat the condition by reducing swelling.

One study of 50 elderly twins found that the twin who used NSAIDs was less likely to get Alzheimer's, or developed it later in life, than the twin who didn't use NSAIDs.

If you are interested in this treatment, talk with your doctor. Don't start taking NSAIDs without his advice. They can cause serious side effects, like stomach irritation and bleeding.

Hormones. New research suggests some hormones may improve your memory. In a recent study, women who took estrogen were one-third less likely to develop Alzheimer's than women who didn't take the hormone. But women aren't the only ones to benefit from a memory-improving hormone. Older men who were given testosterone supplements improved their memories as well.

Vitamin E. Inexpensive and widely available, vitamin E supplements show great promise for slowing down the progress of Alzheimer's disease. In a recent study, people with moderate cases of Alzheimer's were given 2,000 international units (IU) of vitamin E a day. As a result, they were able to care for themselves an average of seven months longer than those who didn't take the vitamin.

A 2,000-IU dose of vitamin E is much larger than the RDA and could cause bleeding problems. Talk with your doctor before taking such large doses.

If you want to get more vitamin E naturally, eat soybeans, green leafy vegetables, wheat germ, whole-grain cereals, peanut butter, nuts, and eggs.

Sugar. A spoonful of sugar helps the medicine go down, according to Mary Poppins. But according to scientific research, a spoonful of sugar may help you remember to take your medicine. In one study, participants fasted overnight. Then, in the morning, they drank lemonade that had been sweetened either with sugar or a sugar substitute. Those who got the lemonade with sugar performed much better at a memory test than those who got the artificial sweetener.

Beta carotene. Keeping your memories may be as simple as crunching some carrots. A recent study found that beta carotene, a substance found in carrots and other brightly colored fruits and vegetables, may help protect you from memory loss and other forms of mental impairment.

Researchers studied more than 5,000 people ages 55 to 95. They found that those whose diets included the most beta carotene were the least likely to have problems with memory, attention span, and other mental abilities.

But if you despise carrots, don't despair. You can also get beta carotene in dark green vegetables, like spinach and broccoli, and in yellow or orange fruits and vegetables, like apricots and sweet potatoes.

Ginkgo. You may be able to leave your memory problems behind with the help of the ginkgo or maidenhair tree, the oldest living species of tree.

Researchers say ginkgo widens your blood vessels, which increases blood flow throughout your body. More blood flowing to your brain means clearer thinking and better memory. Ginkgo has been shown to improve lack of concentration and energy, confusion, absent-mindedness, anxiety, dizziness, and headache.

Although it's still a controversial treatment, several studies show that ginkgo has a positive effect when given to people with Alzheimer's. While it can't reverse the ravages of the disease, taking it may improve thinking, emotional well-being, behavior, and sleeping habits. The studies showed few, if any, side effects.

If you want to try this natural supplement, it's important to choose a good quality extract of ginkgo biloba. Look for the words "50:1 concentrate" and "tannin free" on the label. The 50:1 means that 50 pounds of leaves were used to make one pound of extract, which is the most effective ratio. Tannin free means that tannin, a potentially toxic substance found in the leaves, has been removed during processing.

Amounts used in the studies varied from 120 to 160 milligrams (mg) of ginkgo a day up to 240 mg. For people with Alzheimer's, these large doses seem more effective than the smaller doses you might take to boost memory power.

B vitamins. These vitamins are particularly vital to your brain's health and keeping your memory sharp.

Vitamin B12 (cobalamin) helps your body manufacture neurotransmitters, chemicals that help carry messages between nerves and your brain. If you are a vegetarian, you may need to take supplements, since B12 is only found in foods from animals. Although the recommended dietary allowance (RDA) for B12 is only 2.4 mcg, some memory experts recommend 100 — even 1,000 — mcg daily. Good food sources of vitamin B12 include red meat, salmon, and dairy products.

Vitamin B1 (thiamin) helps nerve signals travel from your brain to different parts of your body. You can get thiamin from wheat germ, nuts, beans, and rice.

• •
Alzheimer's vaccine close at hand

A vaccine to prevent Alzheimer's disease may sound like science fiction, but in a few years, it could be medical fact.

Researchers are busy trying to turn their latest discovery — an enzyme responsible for plaque build-up in the brain — into a new treatment. They are hoping to develop a drug that will block the activity of this enzyme, which might save nerve cells responsible for memory.

In the not-so-distant future, combining tests that accurately predict who will develop Alzheimer's with a vaccine to prevent the disease could mean the end of this tragic condition altogether.
• •

Safeguard your home against accidents

If you are caring for a loved one with dementia or Alzheimer's disease, their safety is your main concern. But because you're dealing with the combination of a childlike mind and an adult body, keeping them safe is not always easy. Like a child, they don't understand danger. Like an adult, they are able to reach, open, close, and use potentially dangerous items.

Protect against household poisons. One of the most dangerous items is probably in your bathroom or kitchen right now — pine oil cleaning solution. Over 10,000 cases of pine oil poisoning are reported each year, making it one of the most common methods of accidental poisoning.

Because it smells and tastes good, people with Alzheimer's are likely to be confused and drink it. It doesn't take much — as little as 8 ounces can be fatal. Although dying from drinking a pine oil cleaner is rare, the elderly are at greater risk because of generally poor health and weakened immune systems. Accident-proof your home against this kind of tragedy by locking away all potentially dangerous substances.

If you suspect someone of accidental pine oil poisoning, check first for a pine aroma on their breath and then get them to a doctor quickly. Other immediate symptoms include headache, blurred vision, dizziness, sluggishness, lack of coordination, sore throat, nausea, vomiting, abdominal pain, and diarrhea.

Fend off falls. As people age from 70 to 80 years old, the number of falls causing severe head injuries nearly doubles. Weaker muscles and joints, poor vision and balance, and certain medications all contribute. But mental conditions, like Alzheimer's, often leave even the most physically fit senior vulnerable to accidents.

Whether you have a short- or long-term guest with Alzheimer's, inspect the inside of your home. Examine the amount of clutter and the placement of extension cords, rugs, pets, and handrails. Be especially mindful of lighting stairways and halls and providing night lights. Outside, check sidewalks, steps, and your driveway for evenness; clear away plants and other natural materials; and provide lights and handrails.

Remember, head injuries only increase the risk of developing further senility.

New ways to help people cope

What do angel fish and salsa music have in common? They are new ideas for comforting and stimulating people with Alzheimer's disease.

Keep a song in your heart. If you want to really light a fire inside someone with Alzheimer's, try a little Tommy Dorsey, Pavarotti, Streisand, or even Willie Nelson.

Studies show that music can improve anybody's awareness, memory, and communication skills. And it's been proven that people with Alzheimer's who listen to music in the evening are less anxious and depressed. Now, researchers at the Department of Psychiatry and Behavioral Sciences at the University of Miami School of Medicine are studying just how this happens.

A small number of male Alzheimer's patients at a veteran's hospital in Florida received half-hour music therapy sessions five mornings a week for four weeks. Blood levels of different hormones were checked before and after therapy.

The interactive therapy involved playing instruments, singing, and drumming. The music included big band, Broadway tunes, spirituals, opera, country and western, and Cuban folk music — whatever was of special interest to the patients. It's important to find out what music sparks a response.

Not only did the therapists and staff notice behavioral changes, but the researchers found hard evidence, as well. The patients:

- learned and sang new songs.

- improved their ability to follow rhythmic patterns.

- were better able to change volume and tempo within the songs.

- recalled endings of phrases and songs.

- became more social — interacting and conversing with others.

The blood tests showed changes, too. Several hormones increased temporarily — just during the four weeks of therapy. However, levels of melatonin, the hormone that regulates sleep patterns, mood, and sexual behavior, stayed higher even six weeks after the experiment.

Researchers know melatonin decreases with age, more so in people with Alzheimer's. And they know over 60 percent of these people suffer from violence, sleep disorders, suicide, depression, and anxiety. If, as this study suggests, music increases melatonin levels, improving many of the behavior problems associated with Alzheimer's could be just a song away.

Fill a tank with tropical fish. Even if someone with Alzheimer's doesn't like to eat fish, looking at fish may help them eat more. That's what Purdue University nursing professor Nancy Edwards discovered at three Indiana nursing homes.

Special aquariums fitted with locked lids; unbreakable glass; and movable, tip-proof stands were placed in nursing homes. The colorful, moving fish immediately interested the people with Alzheimer's. Many would sit and watch the fish for up to half an hour — an unusual behavior for these seniors. Some experienced breakthroughs in communicating and interacting with others, as well as memory. But perhaps most importantly, their eating habits improved.

Good nutrition for people with Alzheimer's is a real concern. Many times, supplements are the only way to ensure they're getting all the necessary vitamins and minerals, even though this is not the healthiest strategy. Amazingly, after the fish tanks were brought in, the 60 people in the study ate up to 21 percent more food.

Try it yourself. By introducing a safe, but stimulating, pastime like this to someone with Alzheimer's, you could improve his diet and quality of life.

Anemia

Sidestep a deadly deficiency

You remember the popular supplement commercials, "Do you have iron-poor blood?" Anemia may seem like a harmless condition, but, unfortunately, it can be a little more complicated and serious than that.

Iron-deficiency anemia can be caused by blood loss, problems with your body's absorption of iron, or not getting enough iron in your diet. However, anemia is sometimes an indication of another problem, especially in elderly people.

A recent study of people over age 85 found that those who were anemic had a death rate twice as high as people the same age with normal blood iron levels. Researchers found that 13 percent of anemic people had cancer during the follow-up period, compared with just 5 percent of the people who were not anemic. Anemics were also more likely to have peptic ulcers and infections.

Another study found that elderly people who were anemic were more likely to have a decline in mental function than those with normal blood iron levels.

While you should strive to get enough vitamins and minerals, including iron, in your diet, deciding to take an iron supplement without your doctor's advice isn't a good idea. Too much iron can be as dangerous as too little, and if you have a problem absorbing iron, taking supplements won't do you any good.

Have your doctor check your iron levels and then follow his advice. In the meantime, here are some suggestions for maintaining a healthy iron level.

Start with some meat. The best food for replacing iron is red meat, particularly organ meats such as calf liver and kidney. The type of iron found in meat, fish, and poultry is more easily absorbed into your body than other types of iron. Here's a good rule of thumb — the darker the meat, the greater the iron content. Dark meats are also rich in vitamin B12 and zinc, important nutrients in preventing anemia.

Pass the peas and beans, please. Since the best natural source of iron is red meat, a strict vegetarian diet can lead to iron deficiency. But with all that fat and cholesterol, you might be shy about loading up on liver. A simple solution to this problem is to eat white poultry with legumes, such as peas or dried beans. Studies show that the animal protein in the poultry helps your body absorb iron from the veggies.

Consider the alternatives. You don't have to eat meat to get your iron. Iron that doesn't come from meat is usually less concentrated and less easily absorbed by your body, but it still helps the fight against anemia. Eggs, dairy products, and grains are good sources of iron. If you're a fan of soy, try tofu or any number of other soy products. Dried fruits, nuts, and blackstrap molasses are also good sources of iron.

Think green and leafy. One of the best ways to make sure you get the iron you need is by eating your green leafies. While green leafy vegetables don't contain much iron, they do contain a lot of folic acid and other nutrients. Folic acid plays a key role in helping your body absorb iron and the equally important vitamin B12.

Juice it up. A tall glass of orange juice is a great way to start the day, but did you know it can also chase away anemia? Vitamin C makes it easier for your body to absorb iron. It is so important, in fact, that a lack of vitamin C can sometimes cause anemia. Some nutrition experts say you should get at least 500 milligrams (mg) of vitamin C every day, while others claim you can safely take up to 20 times that amount. Ask your doctor what's best for you.

•••••••••••••••••••••••••
Unusual warning sign

There's nothing quite like a juicy, home-grown tomato. Yet, if you're eating several of these "love apples" daily, it could be a warning sign of anemia.

In a letter to *The New England Journal of Medicine,* a doctor in Ohio reports that one of his patients came to see him complaining of breathing problems upon exertion and fatigue. She said she craved tomatoes and had eaten six to 10 fresh, whole tomatoes daily for the past two months. When her blood was tested, it revealed low iron levels, and her doctor prescribed iron supplements. When her iron deficiency disappeared, so did her tomato craving.

Cravings aren't uncommon in people with iron deficiency anemia. Up to 58 percent of the cases of iron deficiency anemia are associated with pica, a craving for unusual foods. The most common form of pica is the craving for ice, but some people with pica will eat large amounts of crunchy foods, such as peanuts, celery, or pretzels.

An occasional craving for a particular food is normal, but if your craving persists, ask your doctor to check your iron levels.
••••••••••••••••••••••••

Arthritis

Natural remedies soothe achy joints

Half of the arthritis sufferers polled in a recent survey said they have used alternative therapies because their prescribed medications didn't work. The following natural remedies won't stop your arthritis from getting worse, but they may relieve your pain and improve your quality of life.

Tame your pain with vitamins. Researchers gave a combination of two B vitamins, folic acid (vitamin B9) and cobalamin (vitamin B12), to people with osteoarthritis in their hands. These people had fewer tender joints and as much gripping power as people who took NSAIDs (nonsteroidal anti-inflammatory drugs), such as aspirin or ibuprofen. Their pain did not completely disappear, but it was easily controlled with acetaminophen when necessary. One big benefit of taking B vitamins for arthritis is not suffering any of the side effects of NSAIDs.

At the Boston University Medical Center, 640 people were tested to see if a high intake of vitamin C would help prevent cartilage loss and osteoarthritis of the knee joints. Those who consumed the least vitamin C saw the disease progress three times faster than those with the highest intake. For the people who took in lots of vitamin C, there was also less knee pain. Although natural food sources are best, most experts say it's generally safe to take a supplement.

Doctors researching the role of vitamin D in osteoarthritis think the cartilage in your joints may be protected by this vitamin. They also think vitamin D may actually keep the bones of your joints intact. The bottom line is this — if you have osteoarthritis, make sure you're getting enough vitamin D. Without it, the risk of your arthritis getting worse is three times as great. The best source of this valuable nutrient is sunshine. When you're exposed to sunlight, your body manufactures vitamin D. If you get out in the sun for about 30 minutes every day, you'll get all you need. You can also get vitamin D in fortified milk; boiled shrimp; eggs; and fatty fish, such as salmon, tuna, and sardines. Only take vitamin D supplements under your doctor's care — too much can be toxic.

Rub on a little relief. Researchers have found that capsaicin, the active ingredient in red peppers, is effective in relieving arthritis pain. Made from dried cayenne peppers, capsaicin cream is absorbed through your skin and works by deadening local nerves. Using capsaicin can make exercise less painful, which can help you follow a regular exercise schedule. It can also reduce the amount of other drugs you take.

Many ointments, lotions, and gels contain ingredients that produce a cool or warm feeling on your skin and bring pain relief to your joints. Don't use them for more than a week and never combine them with heating pads or lamps.

Cool it down or heat it up. Many doctors and physical therapists will let you decide whether heat or ice makes your painful joints feel better. Heating pads, gel packs, and even homemade compresses can be very helpful. You can make your own by filling an old sock with rice or salt. Heat in the microwave until it is warm, but not hot, then lay it on your aching joint. For cold relief, put unpopped popcorn kernels into a zip-lock freezer bag. Keep it in the freezer for on-the-spot relief.

Heed the healing power of herbs. According to researchers, using arnica compresses on arthritic joints brings relief from soreness and stiffness because it acts like a painkiller.

To make an arnica compress, dilute a tablespoon of arnica tincture in two cups of water. Soak gauze pads or other absorbent material and apply to the affected area. You can buy arnica tincture at health food stores or pharmacies that sell natural and homeopathic medicines. A word of caution — arnica is for external use only. If taken internally, it is poisonous and can cause elevated blood pressure and cardiac arrest. Also, some people are sensitive to an ingredient in arnica and may develop a rash from using the compress.

Make sure you tell your doctor if you use any form of alternative therapy, whether it is an herb, chiropractic care, exercise, copper bracelets, or vitamins. That will prevent him from prescribing a medication that could possibly interact with one of these remedies.

●●●●●●●●●●●●●●●●●●●●●●●●●●●●
Painful joints? Maybe it's not arthritis

Just because your joints are achy, don't assume you have arthritis. There are other conditions that can trigger joint pain.

Human parvovirus B19. If you're suffering from chronic anemia, sickle cell anemia, AIDS, or another immune system deficiency, you could develop human parvovirus B19, more commonly called chronic arthropathy. This virus can trigger prolonged arthritis pain, as well as a flu-like illness with fever, headache, muscle aches and sometimes nausea, vomiting, or a rash. The arthritis symptoms caused by parvovirus usually go away within a month, but some people will suffer joint pain for several months. If you have this condition, your doctor might recommend a blood transfusion, or he might boost your immune system with gamma globulin, a protein formed in the blood.

Food poisoning. Besides the stomachache, nausea, and diarrhea of food poisoning, *Salmonella* bacteria can also cause joint pain, even weeks after the initial infection. Raw eggs are the most common source of *Salmonella*, but it is also found in raw meats, poultry, dairy products, fish, shrimp, salad dressing, cake mixes, cream-filled desserts, peanut butter, and chocolate. To protect yourself, never eat anything that contains raw eggs, use pasteurized eggs when you can, and cook all meats thoroughly.

Drug side effects. Some prescription drugs cause joint pain as a side effect. If you think your medicine is causing your joint pain, talk with your doctor. Don't stop taking it without his advice.

• •

Put the bite on pain with these foods

The next time you're shopping for groceries, think carefully before you put any food in your cart. Researchers have discovered that what you eat can influence swelling, pain, and stiffness in your joints.

Pick fruits and vegetables. In one study, people with rheumatoid arthritis stayed at a "health farm" for a month. They fasted for a week, then began eating vegetarian diets. The study participants immediately showed improvement — less painful and swollen joints, greater hand strength, and better overall health. Over the course of a year, they gradually added dairy products to their vegetarian diet and continued to improve. The researchers believe several things could have brought on these remarkable changes:

• Foods containing gluten, which is found in wheat and other grains, were completely removed from the eating plan. These are known to make rheumatoid arthritis worse.

• Specific foods that trigger arthritis symptoms, such as food allergies, were eliminated on an individual basis.

• Fatty acids, believed to cause inflammation, were greatly reduced in the vegetarian diet.

- A healthy eating plan battles malnutrition, strengthens your immune system, and makes you less likely to suffer from disease.

- Those on this eating plan lost weight, which can increase your activity level and sense of well-being.

If you want to try a vegetarian diet, make sure you know how to meet your vitamin and mineral needs. Keep in mind that vitamin B12 is only found in foods of animal origin. This means strict vegetarians may become deficient.

Go fish. Eating fish once or twice a week may cut your chances of developing rheumatoid arthritis — but broil or bake it, no frying allowed. Although past studies suggest the omega-3 polyunsaturated fatty acids found in fish oil help control rheumatoid arthritis symptoms, this is the first time researchers found evidence that how you cook your fish can make a difference. Only broiling or baking reduced the risk of rheumatoid arthritis, and adding a third serving of fish each week dramatically increased the protection. Choose salmon, mackerel, brook trout, bluefish, herring, or sardines for this joint-saving benefit.

Sip green tea. Animal studies have shown that green tea, with more antioxidants than most vegetables, may prevent rheumatoid arthritis or at least make the symptoms less severe. Although scientists are looking for more hard evidence in humans, go ahead and brew yourself about four cups of this healthy drink each day — it's a simple, natural way to fight disease.

Walk away from arthritis pain

If you want to keep your joints flexible and strengthen your muscles, get up and get moving. Recent studies show that if you have osteoarthritis in your knees or hips, regular aerobic or weight-training exercises will lessen your pain, improve your walking ability, and boost your health.

The best approach is to balance periods of activity with rest. And vary your routine — switch off between fitness walking, aerobics, water aerobics, weight-lifting, swimming, cross-country skiing, cycling, or dancing. Start slowly, taking care to warm up, and rest joints that are red and inflamed.

A few tools can make your exercise program easier. When you're resting, try using a straight-backed chair instead of a recliner. If your bed is soft, try switching to a firmer mattress. Shoes with good shock-absorbing properties help make walking more comfortable, and a walking stick can reduce the pressure on a painful hip by 20 to 30 percent. Be sure to choose a sturdy wooden or metal stick, with a comfortable handle, that comes to the top of your pelvis. Hold the walking stick on the side opposite your painful joint.

For people who already have arthritis, light aerobic exercise may be better than the more vigorous kind. But researchers are beginning to recognize that for some people, intense, vigorous, aerobic exercise is the therapy that keeps arthritis under control. It can help prevent weight gain, a problem that puts more stress on your joints and makes arthritis worse. In addition, it can improve your overall physical condition, your mental attitude, and your quality of life.

But remember — the wrong type of exercise will increase your risk of developing arthritis or make the condition worse. Watch out for any sport or recreational activity that:

- involves constant shocks to your joints, like basketball or running

- requires you to repeatedly bend your knees, like certain calisthenics

•   means picking up heavy loads, like power-lifting

You may be able to keep arthritis symptoms at bay if you exercise at least three times a week for 30 minutes each time. Talk with your doctor or physical therapist and tailor an exercise program to meet your needs. Besides increasing your strength and improving your health, exercise can give you a feeling of control over your arthritis.

• •
Hot tubs — to soak or not to soak

Hot tubs are a wonderful way to relax and soak away the stresses of your day, but are they good for your arthritis? The Arthritis Foundation suggests knowing the facts before jumping in.

• Warm water causes your blood vessels to dilate. This increases circulation, which improves joint health.

• Gentle exercises in warm water won't damage or stress joints but will provide good resistance to strengthen muscles.

• Water jets provide good massage therapy for tight or sore muscles.

• The warm water will relieve pain and stiffness in arthritic joints, like hot compresses.

• If you have heart disease or a circulatory problem, water that is too hot can put a strain on your heart.

• Talk with your doctor if you have lung disease, high or low blood pressure, multiple sclerosis, diabetes, or any other serious condition.

• If you have had joint replacement, get your doctor's permission before soaking in a hot tub.

• Make sure you can enter and exit the hot tub easily. Put in handrails and nonslip surfaces.

- If you're thinking about buying a hot tub, make sure you can service and maintain it easily — without heavy lifting or risk of falls.

• •

NSAIDs vs. acetaminophen — which pain reliever is best?

According to studies, both acetaminophen and nonsteroidal anti-inflammatory drugs (NSAIDs), like aspirin and ibuprofen, give the same short-term relief from the painful symptoms of osteoarthritis.

But here's something to keep in mind — up to half of the people taking NSAIDs for arthritis will suffer from stomach problems, and many will quit the therapy because of it. Thousands will experience gastrointestinal complications serious enough to require hospitalization and many will die.

Your risk of side effects from NSAIDs is greater if you are elderly, take more than one kind at once, have a history of ulcers or intestinal bleeding, also use corticosteroids or blood-thinners, or suffer from any other serious illness.

Here's how you can prevent damaging your stomach and intestines:

- Take acetaminophen, salsalate, magnesium salicylate, or tramadol instead of NSAIDs.

- Take the NSAID along with another medication designed to protect your stomach from bleeding, like cimetidine or ranitidine. Check with your doctor.

- Get specific instructions on the dose you should take and how long to take it. Unless your doctor says otherwise, don't take any of these pain relievers for more than 10 days.

- Stick with the four nonprescription NSAIDs that fall within the medium-risk category — ibuprofen, ketoprofen, aspirin, or naproxen.

- Fill out a questionnaire developed by a senior research scholar at Stanford University School of Medicine. It estimates your risk of developing gastrointestinal bleeding from taking NSAIDs. You can find the questionnaire, called the Stanford Calculator of Risk for Events (SCORE), on the Internet at <www.seniors.org/score> or ask your doctor for a copy.

- Ask your doctor about celecoxib, a new prescription anti-inflammatory drug. It has been proven to cause fewer ulcers and less stomach bleeding than traditional NSAIDs.

Many doctors now prescribe acetaminophen for their patients with osteoarthritis just to avoid the stomach upset from traditional NSAIDs. Here are a few things to consider:

- Acetaminophen doesn't help reduce inflammation as well as NSAIDs. That can mean less pain relief.

- Make sure your acetaminophen formula doesn't contain caffeine. If arthritis aches and pains are making it difficult for you to sleep, you don't need the added stimulant from caffeine.

- While NSAIDs and acetaminophen give almost equal relief for moderate pain, some experts have found that NSAIDs are more helpful if you suffer severe joint pain.

If you believe your joint pain is caused by arthritis, get a professional diagnosis. Some types of arthritis should not be self-treated, like rheumatoid arthritis, Lyme arthritis, gout, or psoriatic arthritis. If you have osteoarthritis, your doctor will probably recommend over-the-counter medication.

• •

SAMe blasts osteoarthritis

A natural osteoarthritis treatment with a 20-year track record and no side effects sounds too good to be true, but if you've been following the European health trends, you know S-adenosyl-methionine delivers.

Also known as SAM, SAM-e, or SAMe (pronounced sammy), this supplement is well on its way to replacing traditional treatments, like ibuprofen and naproxen, for easing the pain and inflammation of osteoarthritis. But unlike these NSAIDs, SAMe seems to have no serious side effects.

Originally prescribed in Europe to treat depression, doctors noticed this natural compound helped their patients' joint problems.

Researchers have tested 600 to 1,600 milligrams (mg) of SAMe a day to treat osteoarthritis. However, if you plan on taking supplements for your arthritis pain, experts recommend about 200 mg twice a day — and make sure you give the supplements about two months to work.

Since SAMe is sold in the United States only as a nutritional supplement, it is not regulated for quality or ingredients. An independent consumer lab tested 13 SAMe products and only six actually contained what their labels claimed. SAMe is a promising new option if you suffer from osteoarthritis, but for now, it is clearly a case of buyer beware.

• •

Asthma

12 secrets to avoiding attacks

Watch out for acetaminophen. Glutathione, an antioxidant found naturally in your lungs, is thought to prevent your trachea and bronchial tubes from becoming inflamed during an asthma attack. Acetaminophen (Tylenol) uses up this antioxidant, leaving your airways more vulnerable. Research shows a link between people who take acetaminophen frequently — weekly to daily — and severe cases of asthma. If you suffer from asthma and take acetaminophen regularly, check with your doctor.

Stay away from sulfites. In an Australian study, about one-third of the asthma sufferers reported that alcohol, most frequently wine, triggered their asthma attacks. Experts say it's likely the sulfites in wine and other foods are the cause.

Sulfites preserve food and sterilize the bottles used for alcoholic beverages, like wine. Foods high in sulfites are dried fruits, except dark raisins and prunes; bottled lemon and lime juice; beer, wine, and wine coolers; pickled foods; molasses; dried potatoes; sparkling grape juice; wine vinegar; gravy; and maraschino cherries. You'll often find sulfite-treated foods in a salad bar. To avoid sulfites, read food labels in the store and ask at your favorite restaurants.

Consider caffeine. Caffeine can help relieve some asthma attacks by relaxing and expanding the air passages in your lungs — but don't overdo it. Too much caffeine can increase your blood pressure and heart rate and cause insomnia. A moderate amount, especially during an asthma attack, may feel like a breath of fresh air.

Defend yourself with fish oil. A study of Eskimo, Japanese, and Dutch populations links a diet high in omega-3 fatty acids, or fish oil, to low instances of asthma. Small amounts of fish oil over a long period of time seem to give the best results. Good natural sources are mackerel, salmon, striped bass, lake trout, herring, lake whitefish, anchovy, bluefish, and halibut. If you'd like to try fish oil supplements, talk it over with your doctor first.

Boycott processed foods. Much of the food you eat is processed. This means flavorings, preservatives, sweeteners, conditioners, and artificial colors are added to make the products look or taste better and last longer on the shelf. Amazingly, very few people react to the more than 2,000 FDA-approved additives routinely used in food, but there are exceptions. Some people will have an asthma attack after eating food artificially colored with FD&C yellow No. 5. It's used in cake mixes, chewing gum, ice cream, cheese, and soft drinks.

Mind your MSG. Many people think a flavor enhancer called monosodium glutamate (MSG) brings on severe asthma attacks in people sensitive to this additive. For several years, Chinese food received most of the blame for the MSG reaction. Now, however, it may be safe to order your favorite Chinese food once more. Certain studies pointing the finger at MSG turned out to be flawed. The trouble was traced to heartburn, anxiety, depression, or other food allergies. Talk with your doctor to be sure.

Breathe easier with ginkgo. Ginkgo may prevent bronchospasms, a sudden narrowing of the main air passages from the windpipe to the lungs. If you have asthma, a bronchospasm feels like a tightening or squeezing in your chest that makes it difficult to breathe. Ginkgo biloba extract, or GBE, is sold as a food supplement. While no serious side effects have been reported, some people taking ginkgo experience headaches or digestive problems.

Knock off extra pounds. Your weight has a lot to do with how well you breathe. If you have asthma and are clinically obese, losing weight can improve your lung function, decrease your asthma symptoms, and restore your overall health. You may even be able to reduce your medication with your doctor's approval.

Exercise with caution. Part of shedding extra pounds is sticking to an exercise plan. But if you have a condition called exercise-induced asthma (EIA), vigorous activity can set off a chain reaction in your airways that leaves you dizzy, tired, and wheezing. It's a common problem affecting 80 to 90 percent of asthma sufferers. But did you know that eating certain foods even two hours before you exercise can trigger an episode? Shrimp, celery, peanuts, egg whites, almonds, and bananas are the most common causes of food-related EIA attacks. In some cases, the typical asthma symptoms become worse than usual, even resulting in collapse.

Heal your heartburn. You probably never thought heartburn could make it hard to breathe, but researchers have discovered an amazing link between gastroesophageal reflux disease (GERD) and asthma. Studies show up to 80 percent of asthma sufferers also have GERD, a condition where stomach acid backs up into the esophagus, causing heartburn. If your breathing problems didn't start until you were an adult and there's no history of asthma in your family, heartburn could be causing your symptoms. Other signs are wheezing or coughing at night or after exercise or meals. If you treat your reflux disorder, you may find asthma relief at the same time. Talk it over with your doctor and follow his advice.

Give up the gas. If you're cooking with gas, you're twice as likely to develop breathing problems — especially the wheezing and shortness of breath associated with asthma. If you already suffer from asthma, you could be making it worse. Nitrogen dioxide released from gas stoves can irritate respiratory tracts, especially in women, increasing their risk of asthma and serious asthma attacks.

Using an exhaust fan doesn't seem to help since it only removes cooking odors and water vapor, not cooking fumes.

Get out the vacuum. You may hate to do it, but vacuuming every week will help you breathe easier. Studies show there is a big difference in the amount of allergens in a home vacuumed weekly as opposed to monthly.

Breathe easier with remarkable supplement

When you think of algae, you probably picture green scum floating in ponds and lakes. Scientists are now looking at this simple organism as a new, natural treatment for exercise-induced asthma.

If you have this type of asthma, vigorous activity can set off a chain reaction in your airways that leaves you dizzy, tired, and wheezing. It's a common problem for 80 to 90 percent of asthma sufferers.

The specific alga scientists are studying — *Dunaliella salina* — only grows in saltwater ponds in California, Hawaii, and Australia and was first used as a natural food dye. When the European Scientific Committee on Food tested *Dunaliella*, they found it to be nontoxic and a natural source of beta carotene.

Scientists have long argued whether antioxidants, like beta carotene, can help people with asthma. Researchers decided to test a daily dose of this beta carotene-rich alga. They found that 64 milligrams (mg) of *Dunaliella* prevented exercise-induced asthma attacks in over half of the people with asthma.

You can find *Dunaliella* algae supplements in your local health food store or on the Internet. Most producers extract the natural carotenoids, like beta carotene, alpha-carotene, and lutein, from the algae and package it in capsules.

If you're affected by exercise-induced asthma, you might want to give this natural remedy a try. But remember, if you have any undesirable side effects, stop immediately.

• •

Instant relaxation tips calm asthma attacks

Your chest and neck muscles tighten up. You're wheezing and coughing. You can't get a breath.

No matter how long you've lived with asthma, an attack can be scary. It's easy to panic, but that's the worst thing you can do. Rapid and shallow breathing makes the attack worse and can prevent your inhaler from working properly.

Here are some quick, simple things you can do to reduce the anxiety that accompanies an asthma attack. You'll be breathing easier in no time:

- Sit down.

- Breathe deeply and as slowly as possible.

- Squeeze a stress ball.

- Watch fish in an aquarium.

- Sip warm water with a lemon twist.

- Rub a pet.

- Listen to soothing music.

- Look at the sky for one minute.

- Ask a friend to tell you a joke.

• • • • • • • • • • • • • • • • • • • •

Eat your way to better breathing

Researchers say certain vitamins and minerals can improve your asthma symptoms. Although you can take supplements, a healthier alternative is eating foods rich in these nutrients.

Vitamin or mineral	Natural sources
Vitamin C	citrus fruits and juices, strawberries, broccoli, brussels sprouts, sweet red peppers
Vitamin E	baked sweet potatoes, sunflower seeds, fortified cereals
Selenium	liver, kidney, seafood
Magnesium	nuts, legumes, soybeans, seafood, dark green vegetables
Iron	liver, legumes, red meat, shellfish, dried fruit

Maximize inhaler use with these tips

If you suffer from asthma, you probably consider your inhaler your best friend. Here's how you can get the maximum benefits from your asthma inhaler.

Don't combine drugs. Since you use an inhaler for different kinds of asthma medicine — routine drug therapy and emergency treatment — it's very important you don't mix up the two. Using emergency medication on a regular basis can have serious, even fatal, consequences.

Follow instructions carefully. According to a recent study, inhaled corticosteroids are associated with certain kinds of cataracts. Researchers aren't sure why, but they caution people to use their inhalers exactly as instructed.

Get the timing right. Most guidelines tell you to inhale within three to five seconds after releasing the drug. Recent studies now say waiting even two seconds can reduce the amount of medication you actually inhale by 20 percent.

Check with your doctor. Dry powder medications must be inhaled quite vigorously in order to break down large clumps. Children and the elderly, especially those suffering from a severe asthma attack, may not be able to do this properly.

Be consistent. Never interchange medication canisters with different actuators or spacers. Using a different method of dispensing your medication could have serious effects.

Learn proper use. Experts recommend you hold the inhaler one to two inches away from your mouth or use a spacer. If you place the inhaler directly in your mouth, you will inhale more propellant and less medication.

Look for a new type of inhaled asthma drug in the next few years. Researchers at the University of Florida have developed a process that coats each drug particle with a microscopic layer that dissolves over about six hours. The drug is slowly released throughout the day, eliminating the need for continual dosing. The drug will also stay in your lungs rather than being absorbed into your bloodstream where it can cause side effects.

If you follow your doctor's instructions and remember these tips, you'll soon be breathing free and clear.

• •

Beware of royal jelly

You've probably seen royal jelly in your local health food store. It's a natural substance honey bees produce as food for their larvae. While some people claim it can improve your health, boost your energy, and strengthen your immune system, others say it can also mean a sudden, life-threatening asthma attack or allergic reaction.

Many allergists and immunologists think royal jelly contains something that triggers an allergic response in certain people. If you plan to take it, watch out for signs of an allergic reaction — coughing or itching on the roof of your mouth, on your palms, or on your feet.

• •

Back and neck problems

Zap back pain with high-tech breakthrough

If simple chores and pleasures, like bending over to tie your shoes, carrying a bag of groceries, or lifting your grandchild, are causing your back to ache, you might be interested in the latest discoveries about this very common problem.

First, you need to understand some basics of back pain. The older you are when you injure your back, the longer it will take to recover. Experts say if you haven't gotten better in three months, you are unlikely to ever fully mend.

The best solution is to avoid developing back pain in the first place by being careful how you sit, stand, and lift. If you do injure your back, be aware that chronic pain can cause stress, depression, and anxiety. These can make your muscles tight and cramped, making your back pain — and your depression — worse. You can break this painful cycle with relaxation techniques, like yoga, meditation, or visualization.

And finally, use caution if you take pain remedies, especially those containing narcotics. They can cause serious side effects and be habit-forming.

If you're ready to try the latest back-pain remedy, ask your doctor about PENS, percutaneous electrical nerve stimulation. It's a technique based on acupuncture, with a little something extra — electricity.

Doctors insert thin needle probes, similar to acupuncture needles, into the muscles or tissues of your lower back. Then they send a low electrical current through these needles to stimulate the nerves. This stimulation relieves pain and actually allows you to move more freely.

In a recent test, one group of people with chronic low back pain received PENS treatments for 30 minutes, three times a week for three weeks. In this group, 91 percent claimed it was more effective in treating their lower back pain than other pain therapies. They were able to sleep better, took fewer painkillers, and generally had a more positive attitude. They also became more physically active. In fact, PENS therapy looks so promising, doctors are using it to treat the severe pain associated with bone cancer.

Researchers are still trying to establish how often you should receive PENS treatments and how long treatments should last in order to get the best results. But they do recommend you combine PENS with physical therapy and regular exercise. If you don't want to spend another day with an aching back, ask your doctor if PENS is right for you.

●
Beautiful hair can be a pain in the neck

What's your favorite thing about going to the hair salon? If you're like most people, you love getting your hair washed by someone else. And if you're lucky, you'll get a nice scalp massage at the same time. But what about those shampoo bowls? Do you feel as if your neck muscles are twisted and stretched into unnatural positions?

Many doctors would agree with you. In fact, frequent salon shampoos are causing enough chronic neck pain that researchers have given the condition a name — salon sink radiculopathy.

When your neck is frequently pulled and turned, the spinal nerves become damaged and cause pain, not only in your neck but down your arm as well. Your hands and fingers may even feel weak and numb. Researchers believe the chair and sink positions at most hair salons are awkward enough to cause this kind of damage.

To treat this condition, you may have to do specific exercises, take steroids, and even schedule surgery. Better still, avoid it altogether by talking with your hairstylist or the owners of the salon. They should work with you to find a comfortable way to arrange their chairs and shampoo sinks.

●●●●●●●●●●●●●●●●●●●●●●●●

Prolotherapy beats chronic pain

If you suffer from constant pain, a revolutionary treatment called prolotherapy may be the drug-free, nonsurgical answer you're looking for.

Prolotherapy treats musculoskeletal pain, which involves both your muscles and bones. When the tissue that holds your bones together weakens or is damaged, either the bones rub against each other or the neighboring muscles work too hard trying to keep things connected — and that hurts.

A prolotherapist identifies the source of your pain then injects the injured area with natural substances, sometimes along with a small amount of an anesthetic. This alerts your immune system that something is wrong. Blood and nutrients rush to the scene and get busy growing new, healthy tissue. The results are stronger, thicker ligaments that provide better support for your bones and joints. The treatment routine can range from one to eight weeks.

In addition to the injections, prolotherapy endorses a new and different therapy for soft tissue injuries, like sprains — Movement, Exercise, Analgesic, and Treatment (MEAT). Gentle movement and range-of-motion exercises improve blood flow to the area. Natural pain relievers or those that don't decrease inflammation, like acetaminophen, will help you feel better. Prolotherapists believe inflammation is your body's way of curing the problem. They don't recommend taking NSAIDs (non-steroidal anti-inflammatory drugs), like ibuprofen and aspirin, for this type of injury because they decrease swelling.

Treatments like physical therapy, massage, chiropractic care, ultrasound, and electrical stimulation will increase blood flow and cell movement to the injured area. Those who support pro-lotherapy say MEAT allows injuries to completely heal.

Since prolotherapy was first developed in the 1950s, thousands of people have been successfully treated for a wide variety of conditions, such as osteoarthritis, fibromyalgia, migraines, tennis elbow, knee and back injuries, carpal tunnel syndrome, and whiplash.

Prolotherapy is not a cure-all for every kind of pain. That's why it is essential you get an accurate diagnosis and receive treatment from someone trained in prolotherapy. To find a trained prolother-apist in your area, call the American Association of Orthopedic Medicine at 719-475-0032. There are fees for this information.

You can also request a state listing of prolotherapists by send-ing a self-addressed, stamped envelope to: American College of Osteopathic Pain Management & Sclerotherapy (ACOPMS), 5002 E. Woodmill Dr., Wilmington, DE 19808.

Helpful tips to avoid low-back pain

- Try to maintain your spine's normal curves.
- Get a good desk chair and sit straight up; don't slump.
- If you work at a computer, be sure the screen is at eye-level.
- Your chair should support you as you lean forward.

- Don't stay in the same position for very long periods of time.

- Get up and stretch, and walk around every hour or so.

- To lift something from the floor, get close to the object, bend your knees, and bend at your hips. Don't arch your back and stretch.

- When unloading your dishwasher, pivot on your feet so that you keep your hips and shoulders in a line, and bend at the knees and hips.

- To reach a high shelf, put your feet in a staggered stance (one foot in front of the other), then push off your back foot onto your forward foot as you reach up, keeping your hips and shoulders in line.

- To get out of a chair or couch, slide forward to the edge of the seat, and use your legs and arms to lift your body up.

- If you read in bed, place pillows under the small of your back and behind your neck so you can recline, not slump.

Breast cancer

A natural way to fight breast cancer

What you eat — both before and after you are diagnosed with breast cancer — may affect your survival. Here are some ways you can protect yourself from this deadly disease.

Think low fat — not no fat. A low-fat diet can help prevent weight gain, which increases your risk of breast cancer. And cutting the fat in your diet to below 20 percent of your daily calories also lowers your blood estrogen levels. Experts believe less estrogen reduces your risk of breast cancer, but don't go overboard. Your body needs some fat. Here's why:

- It's a great source of energy.

- Your cells need it to function properly.

- It's necessary for human growth.

- Too little fat can cause your cholesterol levels to get worse.

- It carries the fat-soluble vitamins — A, D, E, and K — throughout your body.

The type of fat you eat can play a role in whether you develop breast cancer. A recent study found that monounsaturated fats, found in olive and canola oils, reduced the risk of breast cancer by 45 percent, while polyunsaturated fats, found in corn, safflower, and sunflower oils, increased the risk by 69 percent.

The amount of fat you eat after developing breast cancer may not increase your risk of dying from it. However, if your diet was high in fat before you were diagnosed, you are 70 percent more likely to die from the disease than if you had always eaten low-fat foods.

Drink your milk. Dairy products, especially milk, seem to have a protective effect against breast cancer, even though they are traditionally high in fat. Researchers in Finland studied close to 5,000 women for 25 years. They found the more milk the women drank, the lower their incidence of breast cancer. Even taking into account other factors, like weight, smoking, and diet, the outcome was the same. Other dairy products did not have the same effect. The researchers aren't sure why milk has a protective effect, but they think it may be either lactose or calcium or both.

Steer clear of red meat. Research shows that breast cancer victims who ate the most vegetables and protein — but not red meat — had the highest survival rates. Cutting out red meat and increasing the amount of poultry, fish, dairy, and vegetables you eat may help you survive breast cancer.

● ●
Surprising facts about breast cancer

- A study at Georgetown University Medical Center in Washington, D.C., found that women who are less educated about breast cancer are more likely to be frightened by breast cancer risk counseling and actually have mammograms less often.

- Certain professions may increase your risk of developing breast cancer. In a 20-year study of more than a million women in Sweden, pharmacists, telephone operators, hairdressers, doctors, religious workers, social workers, bank tellers, systems analysts, and computer programmers all had higher percentages of breast cancer than other professions. Although the exact cause is unknown, some experts think the cancer may be related to radiation, electromagnetic fields, or lack of exercise. If you are in a high-risk occupation, monitor your breast health carefully.

- Women at risk of breast cancer are usually more anxious about their breast health and more likely to conduct frequent self-exams. While most experts recommend a monthly self-exam, research shows that many women check their breasts weekly, even daily. This is fine as long as you perform a thorough and careful exam. Frequent, but quick, self-exams are more likely to miss critical changes in breast tissue. So take your time and do it right. If you need guidance, talk with your doctor.

- Find a doctor who will take your symptoms — lumps, pain, nipple discharge, and skin changes — seriously. Studies show that more than 4 percent of women who complain about these symptoms are eventually diagnosed with breast cancer. Even if initial tests come back negative, ongoing symptoms should raise warning flags.

- If you are diagnosed with breast cancer and have a choice, go to a hospital that does a lot of breast cancer surgery. Studies show that your odds of survival are much higher.

• • • • • • • • • • • • • • • • • • • •

Startling cause of men's breast cancer

Breast cancer isn't entirely a woman's disease. Men can get it, too. And now, there's another reason to be concerned. A recent study found that exposure to gasoline fumes can increase a man's risk — and probably a woman's risk as well.

The study looked at men who had held jobs that exposed them to gasoline and combustion products, such as service station attendants and auto mechanics, and compared their rates of breast cancer with other men.

Men who had been exposed to gasoline vapors for at least three months were more than twice as likely to develop the disease as men who hadn't. Men who had held gas-related jobs before age 40 were almost four times as likely to develop breast cancer.

As with any cancer, early detection increases your chances of survival. Although breast cancer is much more common in women, all men should report any breast changes, such as a lump, skin dimpling or puckering; redness or scaliness of the nipple or breast skin; or a discharge from the nipple, to their doctors.

Cancer

Fight cancer at the grocery store

As many as 60 to 70 percent of all cancers could be prevented if people stopped smoking, exercised regularly, and made healthy food choices.

The National Cancer Institute has come up with these dietary guidelines to help prevent cancer.

- Reduce fat intake to 30 percent of calories or less.

- Increase fiber to 20-30 grams a day with an upper limit of 35 grams.

- Include a variety of fruits and vegetables in your daily diet.

- Avoid obesity.

- Consume alcoholic beverages in moderation, if at all.

- Minimize consumption of salt-cured, salt-pickled, and smoked foods.

Besides these general guidelines, researchers have discovered that certain foods may be particularly helpful in preventing cancer.

Fish. Eating fish can improve heart health and increase brain power, but now researchers say it may also help you avoid cancer. Italian researchers divided people with and without cancer into three groups — those who ate fish less than once a week, those who ate about one serving weekly, and those who ate two or more servings a week.

The people who ate two or more servings a week had a much lower risk for certain cancers than those who rarely ate fish. Frequent fish eaters had 30 to 50 percent lower rates of esophageal, stomach, colon, rectal, and pancreatic cancers than people who didn't eat much fish. A high-fish intake was also associated with lower risks for cancers of the larynx, endometrium, and ovaries.

Tangerine juice and orange juice. A high intake of fruit is associated with a lower risk of cancer, and a new study shows that tasty tangerine juice and orange juice contain flavonoids that seem to slow the growth of several types of laboratory-grown human cancer cells.

Tangeretin, a flavonoid found in tangerine juice, was the most effective of the flavonoids studied.

You won't be able to take flavonoids in pill form and expect the same kind of protection. Researchers say synthetic versions of the flavonoids weren't nearly as effective as the real thing, maybe because juices contain other substances that work together to attack cancer cells. Luckily, the real thing is available — healthful and delicious.

Broccoli. Green vegetables are good for you, but when it comes to bladder cancer in men, just a little broccoli can be great. A recent study found that men who ate two half-cup servings of broccoli every week were half as likely to get bladder cancer as men who seldom ate broccoli.

Cut cancer risk in 2 easy steps

Preventing cancer is just one more benefit of a healthy lifestyle. Here are two simple things you can do to dramatically cut your risk of bladder cancer and colon cancer.

Drink lots of water. It's as easy as turning on the tap. If you want to lower your risk of bladder cancer, all you have to do is drink, drink, drink. A 10-year study of almost 50,000 men found that downing just six cups of water each day can cut your risk of bladder cancer in half. Experts believe lots of fluids flush cancer-causing toxins out of your bladder — and your entire body.

Smokers who are at a higher than average risk of developing this dangerous type of cancer can improve their odds, too, just by drinking lots of water.

And if colorectal cancer is a worry for you, drinking water can help. A small study in Taiwan found that men who drank the most water lowered their risk of developing rectal cancer by 92 percent, compared with the men who drank very little water.

Although drinking other liquids will also help, water is the healthiest way to fill your glass.

Maintain a healthy weight. By studying thousands of men and women across the United States, researchers at the National Centers for Disease Control and Prevention found an unmistakable link between obesity and colon cancer.

Some experts believe it's partially due to a substance called prostaglandin E2 (PGE2), an unsaturated fatty acid that helps control the biochemical activity in your tissues. Too much PGE2 increases your risk of colon cancer. If you are overweight or don't exercise, you develop more PGE2. But walking for just an hour a day can decrease the amount of PGE2 in your body by 28 percent.

And then there's the old idea that exercise stimulates your colon and forces partially digested food out more quickly. That would mean potentially harmful or cancer-causing substances don't sit in your intestines where they can cause trouble. The theory is still the same, but scientists think it actually works a bit differently. They now believe your colon slows down its activity during exercise. And then afterward, it increases again, moving food through your intestines even faster.

According to one study, by getting up off the couch and becoming involved in regular physical activity, you've lowered your risk of colon cancer by a whopping 83 percent.

• •
New vaccine may beat prostate cancer

For years, many people have hoped and prayed for a miracle cancer cure. While scientists aren't calling an experimental vaccine a miracle just yet, they are hopeful it will be the beginning of the end for prostate cancer, the second most common type of cancer affecting men in the United States. According to the American Cancer Society, close to 40,000 men will die from it this year.

Cancer researchers at Johns Hopkins Oncology Center and University School of Medicine have developed this vaccine, which uses a powerful "alarm" gene — one that signals your body's entire immune system to recognize and attack cancer cells.

Within four weeks after receiving the vaccination, almost half of the test patients had new immune cells in their bloodstreams fighting their prostate cancer. Although side effects included redness, swelling, and itching around the injection site, none of the patients had to be hospitalized during this experimental therapy.

While the tests were done on men with prostate cancer, the researchers hope eventually this type of vaccination will help your body destroy other cancer cells left behind after traditional treatments, like surgery, chemotherapy, and radiation.

Other cancer vaccines are making big news, as well, but they aren't all miracles either. Although an experimental vaccine for colon cancer may not cure the disease, researchers think it helps gauge how well your immune system is fighting the cancer. They hope giving the vaccine many times over a longer period of time will have more useful results than what they've seen so far.

• •

Catch the latest skin protection tips

Skin cancer is the most common cancer in the United States. To protect yourself, spend less time in the sun, which will reduce your exposure to Ultraviolet (UV) radiation; avoid sunburns, especially if you're young; and check yourself regularly for early signs of skin cancer.

Here are more tips to help keep your skin healthy.

Know your UV Index. There are many factors that can influence how quickly you will burn or damage your skin, including your skin type, distance you are from the equator, the time of year, and the cloud cover. Did you know up to 80 percent of UV radiation can pass through clouds? To help you determine your risk of sunburn, the National Weather Service reports a daily UV Index for 58 different cities around the country. This gives your risk of sunburn within 30 miles of these particular areas. The numbers indicate how much UV radiation reaches the earth in one hour around noon.

You can get your nearest UV Index by calling the EPA Hotline at 1–800–296–1996 or by checking the Internet at <http://www.epa/gov/ozone>.

Weather Service UV Index

UV Index	UV Exposure
0 – 2	minimal
3 – 4	low
5 – 6	moderate
7 – 8	high
9 – 10+	very high

Decide not to tan. The FDA and the American Academy of Dermatology are working together to discourage people from using tanning beds. These two organizations have developed very specific guidelines for tanning bed manufacturers, covering issues like timers, labels, and tanning instructions.

For instance, the beds must:

- use only certain bulbs

- carry warning labels and a tanning schedule

- have an emergency stop control

- include protective eyewear

If you use a tanning bed, the FDA and the American Academy of Dermatology urge you to follow all safety precautions carefully.

Think polyester. For maximum sun protection, select clothing that is heavy or tightly woven. Double-knit polyester has one of the highest sun protection factors. Wool jersey, plain polyester, and polyester/cotton blends are also protective. And although light-colored material is cooler because it reflects heat, experts have found that dyed fabrics have more UV protection than white fabrics. In fact, dark blue material is three times more protective than white.

At least one manufacturer has taken sun protection seriously and developed a line of clothing that blocks UV rays by combining special fibers, tight weaving, and thicker fabric. The company's claims are backed up with solid research. A study at Morehouse School of Medicine shows that this fabric, called Solumbra, protects your skin from the sun's damaging rays better than ordinary fabric. In fact, the FDA has given the manufacturer, Sun Precautions, Inc., of Seattle, Wash., special permission to market their products as "sun protective" with an SPF (Sun Protection Factor) of 30.

You can contact Sun Precautions, Inc., by calling 1–800–882–7860 or 1–888–SOLUMBRA. They also have information and products listed on their Web site <www.solumbra.com>.

Examine your skin. Nearly all skin cancers can be cured if found early, and many growths can be removed in your doctor's office. Visit your doctor for a thorough inspection once a year, especially if you are light-skinned. Between professional exams, get in the habit of checking yourself once a month. You are looking for anything new, like a change in a mole or new growths. Be especially alert for any moles that are unusually shaped, have rough edges or mixed colors, or are larger than a pencil eraser.

Here's a good plan to follow:

- Look at both sides of your hands and at your lower and upper arms.

- Undress completely and stand in front of a full-length mirror. Look at your whole body, front and back. Raise your arms so you can check under them. Use a hand mirror for any back parts you can't see.

- Use the hand mirror to examine your scalp, ears, and the back of your neck. Part your hair or use a blow dryer for a closer look.

- Check out the backs of your legs and the bottoms of your feet with the mirror. Look between your toes, too.

● ●
Compute your need to shun the sun

Take this quick quiz to see if you're at risk of developing skin cancer.

- Do you have red or blonde hair?

- Are your eyes either blue, green, or hazel?

- Do you sunburn easily?

- Do you freckle easily?

- Do you have lots of moles?

- Are you descended from northern European ancestors?

- Have you had several blistering sunburns in your life?

- Were you severely sunburned as a child or young adult?

- Do you live in an area with high solar radiation?

- Do you work or spend most of your time outside?

- Do you use a sunlamp or tanning bed?

If you answered "YES" to eight or more of these questions, consider yourself at high risk of developing skin cancer.

No matter what your score, always use sunscreen; avoid outside activities between 10 a.m. and 2 p.m.; and wear sunglasses, protective clothing, and a wide-brimmed hat.

• •

Salty snacks boost cancer risk

Gone are the days of popping open a can of mixed nuts and munching to your heart's content. You already know salty, fatty snacks aren't exactly healthy eating. But did you know that even a rare indulgence in salty snacks — only twice a month — is enough to almost double your risk of stomach cancer.

Results of a study in Mexico confirm that salty snacks and cured and pickled foods just aren't stomach friendly. Researchers know that salt irritates the stomach lining, and irritation can set the stage for inflammation and eventually cancer. But this new finding is enough to make anyone put down that can of peanuts and think again.

If you can't stand the thought of life without a handful of salty pretzels once in a while, snack away. Just remember to also graze on beans, yellow and orange vegetables, or high-fiber breads and grains twice a day to undo the damage.

Here's how you can lower your risk of stomach cancer:

- Eat more fruits and veggies. Choose ones that are high in vitamin C, a powerful antioxidant cancer fighter. Sweet red peppers and green peppers, citrus fruits, and strawberries are loaded with vitamin C.

- Pick healthier forms of protein. Choose eggs, beans, tofu, miso, and unsalted nuts over salted or smoked meats.

- Develop a taste for green tea. Its powerful antioxidant punch can protect you from cancer and heart disease.

- Jazz up your recipes with spices. Turmeric, the main ingredient in curry, is another antioxidant that also kills bacteria.

- Eat more garlic. Italian and Chinese studies show that garlic and its cousins — onions, leeks, shallots, and chives — all protect against stomach cancer.

Smokers: Beware of these supplements

If you smoke, don't take beta carotene supplements. At least that's what researchers at the University of Texas Medical Branch are saying. Surprising news, considering experts have long considered antioxidants, like beta carotene, to be your body's first line of defense against cancer-causing free radicals. But a new study suggests beta carotene supplements may actually increase a smoker's risk of developing lung cancer.

In animal tests, beta carotene supplements increased the cancer-causing activity of cigarette smoke. When people were tested, heavy smokers taking beta carotene supplements had higher rates of lung cancer and lung cancer-related death.

This means when you smoke and take beta carotene supplements, the carcinogens in the cigarettes are even more active and dangerous, increasing your risk of cancer.

You may think this goes against everything you know about antioxidants and good health, but that's not so. The problem is people have forgotten that getting antioxidants from whole foods is different from taking supplements.

If you're thinking of loading up on antioxidant supplements to fight cancer or other diseases, think again — especially if you smoke. Instead, get your antioxidants from whole foods. The following is a list of foods containing antioxidants, like alpha-carotene; beta carotene; lutein; lycopene; and vitamins A, C, and E.

carrots	sweet potatoes	apricots	tomatoes
spinach	broccoli	mango	cantaloupe
watermelon	cress leaf	collard greens	parsley
pumpkin	meat	dairy	citrus
nuts	peppers	wheat germ oil	sunflower seeds

• •
Don't ignore these warning signs

If you have any of these unusual symptoms, see your doctor.

Waxy, yellow blisters on your eyelids. These could mean trouble somewhere else in your body. Called amyloid deposits, these blisters can grow in almost any organ and can indicate the presence of multiple myeloma, a type of bone cancer.

Headaches. If you suffer from headaches during exercise that go away when you rest, it may be a sign of heart disease. Even if you don't suffer any of the other usual signs of heart problems, be especially alert if you have other risk factors, such as high blood pressure, a history of smoking, or heart disease in your family.

Although the exact link between headaches and heart disease is still unknown, experts caution against ignoring this warning sign.

Seeing spots and flashes of light. This could mean you have a detached retina. That's when your retina has torn or separated from the rest of your eye. You won't feel pain when this happens, but you can suddenly lose your vision. See a doctor immediately so he can surgically reattach it.

A sore on your leg that won't heal, bleeding gums, or a recurring bladder infection. They may seem like harmless ailments, but they are also little-known symptoms of noninsulin dependent diabetes mellitus, more commonly known as Type 2 diabetes. Ask your doctor to run some tests if you are at risk of developing this disease.

- over 40 years old

- overweight

- eat high-fat foods

- inactive

- have a family history of diabetes

- African-American, Hispanic-American, Asian or Pacific Islander, or Native American

• • • • • • • • • • • • • • • • • • •

'Secret' weapon helps defeat cancer

The tests come back positive — it's cancer. But if you have a strong and active faith, you already possess a powerful, secret weapon to fight this deadly disease. Doctors once thought spirituality and religion didn't help much in coping with serious illnesses, like cancer. Now, many experts can't argue with hard scientific research that proves otherwise.

If you participate in organized religion, you are more likely to have a strong support network, better overall mental health, and positive ways of coping with stress or illness. This can be very important when you're dealing with the hopelessness and helplessness of a life-threatening disease. People with strong religious and spiritual beliefs seem better able to face their illness with a positive outlook — coping with it rather than surrendering to it. You are also less likely to become depressed and react to misfortune by drinking, smoking, or participating in other destructive behaviors.

Some of the proven benefits of attending church regularly include less depression and anxiety, a stronger immune system, and lower blood pressure. In fact, the health effects are as positive as not smoking.

You can also benefit even if you aren't ill. Experts say going to church may help you live longer. One research team found you could add seven years to your life by attending church more than once a week. Several studies that followed older adults for up to 30 years saw health benefits for women, in particular, when they attended regular religious services.

Of course, just because you are a religious person doesn't mean you won't get sick. It just means you may be able to better handle the emotional stress of an illness and, perhaps, recover more quickly.

Chronic fatigue syndrome

6 ways to overcome chronic fatigue

No one is sure what causes Chronic Fatigue and Immune Dysfunction Syndrome (CFIDS) — and that makes it difficult to treat. Although some lucky people find their symptoms disappear on their own after a few months, for others, the battle with fatigue rages on and off for years.

While researchers continue to search for a cure, don't let chronic fatigue zap your energy and take over your life. Here are some ways you can fight back:

Get some exercise. Some days you may have more energy than others. When this happens, don't overdo it. You'll probably pay for this overexertion tomorrow with sore muscles and even more fatigue. Even though exercise can help the symptoms of CFIDS, you need to exercise a little restraint as well. And on days when you're tired, do some mild exercises. Ask your doctor to help you choose exercises that are appropriate for your abilities and energy level.

Choose the right foods. While there is no magical eating plan for people with CFIDS, a few dietary guidelines may help you become more energized. Eat plenty of complex carbohydrates, like fruits, vegetables, and whole grains. Many people with CFIDS are prone to allergies, so identify foods you may be sensitive to and avoid them. You should also avoid or limit your intake of alcohol, caffeine, sugar, nicotine, and the artificial sweetener aspartame (Nutrasweet).

Boost your energy with vitamins. When you are ill for a long time, your body often uses up extra amounts of vitamins, creating a deficiency. This could be the case in CFIDS. A multi-vitamin supplement may provide you with the extra vitamins you need, especially the B vitamins, which help your body turn protein and other nutrients into energy.

Lighten your load with lysine. This amino acid supplement is used to help clear up cold sores caused by the herpes virus. It may prevent your body from absorbing another amino acid called arginine, which helps the herpes virus reproduce. Since most people with CFIDS carry some form of the herpes virus, lysine may control the virus and make you feel better. The recommended dosage is 1 to 2 grams of lysine daily. If you decide to take lysine supplements, be sure to avoid foods containing arginine, such as nuts, chocolate, raisins, whole wheat, brown rice, and cereal. These will work against your efforts to control the herpes virus.

Find support. CFIDS can be draining, not only physically but emotionally, too. Contact local support groups, try some counseling, or just lean on your family and friends. Because this disease is so difficult to diagnose, many people need to be reassured that their illness is not "just in their heads."

Keep a journal. Write your daily activities and note the times you seem to have the most energy. If you have peaks and valleys of fatigue at regular times, you may be able to plan your day around the times when you are most likely to be feeling well.

Despite researchers' efforts, chronic fatigue is still a mysterious illness. But as the syndrome affects more and more people, the chances are greater that researchers will find a cause and a cure. In the meantime, take heart in knowing you are not alone, and if others have found a way to live with chronic fatigue, so can you.

● ●

Are you at risk?

The media labeled Chronic Fatigue and Immune Dysfunction Syndrome (CFIDS) the "yuppie flu" a few years ago because most reported cases involved well-educated, middle-class women. New research has better defined exactly who gets this frustrating illness.

Statistics show women are still more likely to suffer from CFIDS than men. If you compare the numbers of women afflicted with various diseases, CFIDS is more common than AIDS, breast cancer, and lung cancer. Although not life-threatening, this makes it one of the least understood but most serious health concerns for women.

CFIDS does not seem to be related to aging, but it strikes more frequently during middle age. This puts the large baby-boom segment of the population at particular risk. Oddly enough, young adults and seniors seem least likely to suffer from this illness.

Clerical workers, salespersons, craftsmen, laborers, and machine operators are more commonly affected than people in professional occupations.

And your risk is higher if you are unemployed, receiving disability income, or working part-time.

● ●

New hope for this frustrating syndrome

Because it's difficult to diagnose, Chronic Fatigue and Immune Dysfunction Syndrome (CFIDS) usually means frustration for both the patient and the doctor.

To make matters worse, many people once thought it was not a real illness. Now experts think about 1 to 4 percent of the population suffer from it, and it's very possible the actual numbers are much higher. If you are faced with a CFIDS diagnosis, you will discover it significantly affects your work and your family life.

Symptoms of CFIDS can include crippling fatigue — weariness so bone-deep you don't want to even get out of bed, flu-like symptoms, infections, muscle pain, weakness, fever, sore throat, headache, joint pain, sleep problems, changes in lymph nodes, confusion, and concentration problems.

Because these symptoms mimic many different conditions and because the main symptom, fatigue, is common in several other illnesses, be sure to rule out these possibilities before you begin any treatment:

- diabetes

- liver problems

- Addison's disease

- congestive heart failure

- anemia

- hyperthyroidism (Graves' disease)

- hypothyroidism

- mononucleosis

CFIDS often begins after you have had an infection, like a cold, bronchitis, or mononucleosis, or after a period of stress or trauma. No one knows for sure what causes it, but a virus, like herpes or the Epstein-Barr virus, or an autoimmune disorder may set it off.

But there's hope. For the first time in their history, the Food and Drug Administration (FDA) authorized testing a nutritional supplement to treat this medical condition. The supplement is called NADH, and the results are amazing.

NADH stands for nicotinamide adenine dinucleotide plus high-energy hydrogen. Never mind that — just remember it's a co-enzyme, a natural substance found in all living cells. Its purpose is to supply your cells with energy. The more you have, the more energetic your cells are. Without enough, your brain and muscle cells can't function properly. Recently, scientists began to explore the idea that supplying your body with more NADH could raise your energy level.

A small study at Georgetown University School of Medicine in Washington, D.C., found that about one-third of people suffering with CFIDS were helped by 10 milligrams of NADH daily. These results so encouraged the researchers that they offered NADH supplements to all the participants in a follow-up study. Positive response to the NADH jumped to an amazing 72 percent — and there were no negative side effects.

Other tests in Europe have had similarly encouraging results. NADH supplements gave people with CFIDS more energy, endurance, and strength. It's also being tested as a possible treatment for Alzheimer's, Parkinson's Disease, and high blood pressure.

You can find NADH supplements in health food stores and on the Internet. It's currently marketed as a nutritional supplement under the brand name Enada, but it may soon be officially named a vitamin by the FDA.

Colds and flu

10 ways to survive the cold and flu season

Here are some simple tips for avoiding colds and flu — and for feeling better fast if you get sick anyway.

Sidestep stress. When you're under stress, your immune system doesn't work as well as it should. This makes your body more vulnerable to infections, including colds and flu. Try to get a handle on your problems by keeping your sense of humor and a healthy perspective. Eliminate the unimportant things in your life. Make time for the people and activities you really care about.

Wash your hands. You can catch a cold or the flu by touching something exposed to the virus, like someone's hand, a telephone, or another surface, then touching your eyes, nose, or mouth. Once germs get into your respiratory system, they'll spread quickly. You can also become infected by inhaling particles in the air from a cough or sneeze. To reduce your chances of getting sick, keep your hands away from your eyes, nose, and mouth, and wash them frequently. Use plain, liquid soap and rub your hands together vigorously for best results. Liquid soap is a better choice because bar soap can harbor germs. The popular antibacterial soaps don't provide protection against colds and flu because they only kill bacteria, not viruses.

Catch extra shut-eye. When your body is working to fight off a cold or the flu, it needs plenty of rest. Don't push yourself. Take a day off from your normal activities. It will help you get well, and it might protect your friends and co-workers from catching your germs.

Bid germs farewell. Keep your house really clean and germ free, and you'll protect yourself from colds and flu. Use a disinfectant, like Lysol, or a solution of bleach and water to clean kitchen counters, doorknobs, cabinet handles, staircase railings, telephones, and anything else you touch. Change pillowcases and hand towels often.

Calm your cough. Make your own natural cough syrup by mixing the juice of one lemon with two tablespoons of glycerine and 12 teaspoons of honey. Take one teaspoon every half hour, stirring before each use. For another soothing and tasty cough reliever, combine 8 ounces of warm pineapple juice and two teaspoons of honey.

Gargle. The best and most comforting gargle for your sore throat is warm, salty water. One-half teaspoon of salt stirred into a cup of warm water will make a soothing solution. Another good gargle is strong, brewed tea, which has an astringent, or drying, effect. You can gargle with it warm or cold.

Get steamed up. If a stuffy nose is making you miserable, try a little steam. The hot, moist air can temporarily clear clogged nasal passages and help you breathe easier. It also can prevent your sinuses from becoming dry and irritated, which could lead to swelling and infection. So jump in the shower, plug in a humidifier, or make your own private steam bath with boiling water in a bowl. Just cover your head with a towel, lean over the bowl, and breathe deeply. Add some chamomile flowers to the water to help clear clogged sinuses, calm your cough, and soothe your irritated throat. Add pine oil, eucalyptus, or menthol for a little extra nasal-opening power. If you can't slow down long enough to sit over a bowl, try this clever home remedy. Cut a strip from the bottom of an old T-shirt. Soak it in hot water or microwave the damp shirt until it's warm. Tie it around your head, covering your nose. This gives you the same effect as sitting over a bowl of hot water, but it allows you the freedom to move around.

Sip some soup. Chicken soup is the classic mother's remedy for colds and flu, and research shows that mom was right on the mark. One study found that even when chicken soup was diluted 200 times, it still interfered with the substances that trigger colds. Other studies found that hot soup can break up congestion and thin out mucous secretions.

Keep your nose clean. A nasal wash or nasal irrigation is an excellent tool for fighting a cold or the flu. It washes bacteria and excess mucus from your sinuses and helps prevent a sinus infection. You'll need a large rubber syringe that you can buy at your local drugstore. Make a solution of one-half teaspoon of plain (not iodized) salt and a pinch of baking soda mixed with one cup of warm water. Fill the syringe, then place it in one nostril and pinch the nostril closed around it. Squeeze the syringe to move the saline solution through your nose, then blow your nose gently. Most of the salty solution will come out through your mouth, so just rinse with plain water to remove it. Continue until the drainage is clean, then repeat with the other nostril. To keep your nasal syringe from reinfecting you later, clean it well after every use. Store it on end in a clean glass so any remaining water can drain out. Don't share syringes. Make sure every family member has his own.

Give hankies the heave-ho. With a cold or flu, you'll probably blow your nose a lot. Be sure to use disposable tissues instead of handkerchiefs. Then you won't reinfect yourself as you're getting well, and you're less likely to infect others. Dispose of dirty tissues carefully in a sealed bag.

Natural ways to relieve symptoms and boost immunity

If you have a cold or the flu, antibiotics won't chase it away. They kill bacteria, not viruses. Nevertheless, there are lots of things you can do to relieve your symptoms and strengthen your immune system. Just remember, before you begin self-treating, make sure you really have a cold or the flu. Rule out other conditions, like *Strep* throat, hay fever, or other allergies that require different treatments.

Fluids. It's very important to drink plenty of fluids when you have a cold or the flu, particularly if you have a fever. To prevent dehydration and to thin the mucus in your lungs so you can cough it up, drink at least eight to 10 cups of liquids every day.

Garlic. Garlic helps fight infections caused by bacteria and viruses, can lower a fever, and is full of the antioxidant vitamins A and C. In a recent study, Boston University medical school researchers claimed garlic works like an antibiotic against *Strep*, *Staph*, and fungus and yeast infections, as well as numerous strains of the flu. If you've got a cold or the flu, experts suggest eating garlic or taking a garlic supplement every day.

Ginger. Soothing a sore throat can be a snap with ginger. For centuries, this herb has battled several illnesses, including colds and the flu, and it may be particularly helpful in reducing mucus. To make a pot of comforting ginger tea, place three or four slices of the fresh root in a pint of hot water. Simmer for 10 to 30 minutes, and sip on the soothing concoction all day.

Vitamin C. At the first sign of sniffles, many people reach for vitamin C. While most experts don't believe it will prevent a cold, they say it may ease symptoms and help you get well faster. What nobody can seem to agree on is exactly how much vitamin C you should take.

The Recommended Dietary Allowance (RDA) for vitamin C is 60 milligrams (mg) a day. In a recent study, researchers gave at least 3,000 mg a day to study participants and found it dramatically reduced cold and flu symptoms. A word of caution — because of possible side effects, check with your doctor before taking large doses of any vitamin. Vitamin C is easy to get naturally by eating sweet red peppers, green peppers, citrus fruits, and strawberries.

Vitamin A. Vitamin A helps keep your immune system healthy so you can fight off infections. The active form of vitamin A is found only in animal sources, like meat and dairy products. However, beta carotene, which is converted into vitamin A in your body, is found in brightly colored vegetables, like carrots, sweet potatoes, spinach, and broccoli. The RDA for vitamin A is 800 micrograms (mcg) for women and 1,000 mcg for men.

Too much vitamin A can be toxic. Fortunately, it is difficult to get too much from food sources. If you take a vitamin A supplement, many nutritionists warn against exceeding the RDA.

Zinc. Taking zinc for a cold is still controversial. In laboratory tests, zinc stops cold viruses from multiplying, but in trials on people, the results are less definite. Some studies have found that people who use zinc gluconate lozenges recover from their colds more quickly than others. Other studies haven't shown any benefits. But researchers agree on one thing — if zinc is to help at all, you must begin using it at the first sign of cold symptoms.

If you want to try zinc, keep these tips in mind. Dissolve zinc lozenges or lollipops slowly. Don't bite or chew them. You need to produce saliva in order for the zinc to help your throat. You may also have mild side effects, especially nausea or a bad taste in your mouth. It may help to take zinc after eating, when your stomach is not empty. It's possible to get too much zinc, which can cause other problems. Take it only for the short period of time you have cold symptoms.

Because of the controversy surrounding zinc's safety and effectiveness, talk with your doctor before taking more than 50 mg a day. People with Alzheimer's disease or those at risk of developing it should avoid zinc supplements.

Echinacea. Native Americans have used this herb for hundreds of years to treat colds, coughs, sore throats, toothaches, and even snakebites. It seems to fight colds and flu by boosting your immune system and, best of all, it has no side effects. Most modern experts agree it is helpful in treating the early stages of upper respiratory tract infections. However, there is no strong evidence it will help prevent them.

You may have trouble deciding which Echinacea product to use since even the clinical trials tested different doses, different species of Echinacea, different types of preparations, and sometimes a combination of herbal products. The well-respected German commission E recommends 300 to 400 mg of dry Echinacea extract three times a day.

Other herbal remedies used to fight colds include marshmallow root, slippery elm, mullein flower, licorice, elderberry, astragalus root, goldenseal root, wild cherry bark (tea or tincture), eucalyptus or camphor rub, honey and lemon, thyme, fenugreek, cayenne, and horseradish.

● ●
Fight flu with elderberries

The tart berries of the elder tree are thought to help heal a variety of respiratory ailments, including colds, flu, asthma, fever, and sore throat. And scientific research is beginning to show that this herbal remedy may really be effective against the flu.

During an outbreak of influenza B in Panama, researchers gave some flu sufferers a standardized elderberry extract. Within two days, about 93 percent of the people who received the extract experienced a significant improvement in symptoms, including fever, while the people who received a placebo didn't show improvements for six days.

Side effects from elderberries are uncommon. So, the next time that achy flu bug strikes, maybe you should give some elderberry extract a try.

• •

A guide to exercising when you're sick

Your nose is stuffy, your throat is raw, and that nagging headache won't go away. Is it best to curl up with a blanket and let your cold run its course, or should you enjoy a morning walk and a game of tennis?

Check your neck. To find out if you should lace up your walking shoes or crawl back into bed, do a neck check. If your symptoms are above the neck — affecting your nose, throat, eyes, or sinuses — go ahead and take part in moderate exercise. This may actually clear your head and help you sleep better. Just gauge how much and how long you exercise by how you feel after the first few minutes. If a few days of easy exercise leaves you feeling depressed and tired, with sore muscles and less energy, you're probably working yourself too hard.

If you are suffering from "below-the-neck" symptoms, like chills, fever, stomach upset, diarrhea, joint or muscle pain, body aches, or a cough, let your body rest. Pushing yourself to work out under these conditions could make you more tired and cause dehydration. And things could get worse. Some medications keep your body from sweating, increasing your risk of heatstroke. Researchers found that if you have a virus in your bloodstream and still exercise vigorously, you increase your chances of developing a critical heart condition called myocarditis.

Keep yourself fit. It's already been proven that keeping fit can help you avoid colds in the first place. Moderate exercise on a regular basis actually strengthens your immune system, making you less vulnerable to the common cold. Exercise stimulates white blood cells called macrophages in your immune system. These "natural killer cells" circulate throughout your body fighting invaders, like viruses and bacteria.

And remember, it's never too late to get started. The older you are, the more you benefit from being in good physical shape. Women over 67 who walk or exercise regularly have fewer respiratory infections than others.

Take it easy. On the other hand, vigorous training can suppress your immune system for days, increasing your risk of an upper respiratory tract infection. One study found that marathon runners were at their highest risk of coming down with a respiratory infection during the two weeks after they raced.

How does this happen? One explanation is that your body is built to protect itself from invaders, like bacteria and viruses, and mucus is its first line of defense. Because viruses are usually airborne, how you breathe partly determines if a virus survives inside your body. If you breathe through your nose, the virus particles are trapped in the mucus at the back of your throat where they can't do any harm.

When you exercise heavily, you breathe faster and through your mouth. More air moves into your air passages and the mucus dries out, making it unable to trap any viruses. They enter your lungs and infect your body.

Researchers say strenuous sports, like rowing and distance or marathon running, can cause more respiratory infections than walking and gentler exercises.

• •
Shot in the arm may protect your heart

Getting a flu vaccine could protect you from more than the flu. It may also lower your risk of heart attack if you have heart disease.

Researchers studying 233 people with heart disease found that those who received a flu shot had a 67 percent lower risk of heart attack.

The researchers aren't sure what might account for this heart-protective effect, but they say heart attacks are more common in the winter months, and tend to be more severe than in warmer weather.

Although more research is needed, check with your doctor about getting a yearly flu vaccine if you have heart disease.

• •

New flu vaccine recommendation

The American Academy of Family Physicians (AAFP) recommends that everyone age 50 and older get a yearly flu shot. They suggested lowering the age from 65 to 50 because the fatality rate from influenza is higher than most people think.

Each year, an estimated 20,000 people die from flu and related complications. During particularly bad outbreaks, the death rate can rise even higher. In 1957 to 1958, the "Asian flu" was responsible for 70,000 deaths in the United States. The worst outbreak of flu occurred in 1918 to 1919 when the "Spanish flu" was responsible for 500,000 deaths in the United States and 20 million deaths worldwide.

Older people aren't the only ones who are susceptible to influenza. The AAFP also recommends that anyone with a chronic disease, such as diabetes or asthma, get a yearly flu vaccine.

Even people who don't fall into the recommended groups can benefit from a flu vaccine. When flu strikes, the cost of time away from work, doctor's visits, and other expenses add up. Cost savings in working adults is an estimated $46.85 per person vaccinated.

Unlike some vaccines that last a lifetime, you have to get a flu shot every year. Flu viruses are constantly mutating, and the immunity you receive from your shot declines over time.

Side effects from flu vaccines are rare. According to the Centers for Disease Control, less than one-third of those who receive the vaccine have some soreness at the vaccination site. About 5 to 10 percent experience mild side effects, such as headache or low-grade fever for about a day after vaccination. In the past, side effects were more common because of impurities in the vaccines, but modern manufacturing techniques have elimi-nated that problem.

People who have a severe allergy to eggs shouldn't get flu vac-cinations. The viruses used in the vaccine are grown in hens' eggs and can cause a serious allergic reaction in those people.

• •
New drug helps prevent flu

Although doctors say a yearly vaccination is the best way to pro-tect yourself from the flu, a new drug is available that may also help.

The drug, oseltamivir, is taken by mouth once or twice daily for six weeks. Researchers say the drug is helpful if a vaccine isn't available or as added protection for people at high risk. It might also be useful in preventing the spread of flu among groups of people who have been exposed to the virus, like people in nursing homes.
• •

Colon cancer

4 ways to beat this deadly disease

Colorectal cancer often begins quietly, with constipation as its only symptom — but don't underestimate it. This deadly disease is the second leading cancer killer in the United States, and the third most common cancer.

Most cases of colorectal cancer begin with the growth of polyps in the colon. These polyps are common, especially in older people, and they are not always cancerous. Nevertheless, researchers estimate that up to 80 percent of colon cancer deaths could be prevented by removing precancerous polyps quickly.

Since symptoms aren't always noticed early, screening for colon cancer is very important, especially if you're at high risk. Risk factors include a family or personal history of the disease; having a colon or bowel disorder, such as irritable bowel syndrome or colitis; having had ovarian, endometrial, or breast cancer; and eating a diet high in animal fat and low in fiber. Your chances of getting colorectal cancer also rise as you age. Many cancer organizations recommend regular screening after age 50.

Eat a high-fiber, low-fat diet. A couple of recent studies have found no evidence that a high intake of fruits, vegetables, and fiber reduces the occurrence of colon polyps in people who already had polyps. However, the studies lasted only a few years, and they may not have been long enough for the protective effect of diet to show up. The bulk of evidence still suggests that a diet low in fat and high in fruits, vegetables, and fiber can reduce your risk of colon cancer, as well as other diseases, such as heart disease, diabetes, high blood pressure, and obesity.

Choose colorful foods. Eating plenty of fruits and vegetables is important to a healthy diet, and when it comes to cancer prevention, color may be the key. A recent study found that fruits and vegetables containing lutein, a kind of carotenoid, may help prevent colon cancer. Carotenoids are substances that give fruits and vegetables their color. Foods high in lutein include spinach, tomatoes, corn, broccoli, oranges, green beans, lettuce, cabbage, and kale.

Ask your doctor about aspirin. Daily aspirin therapy has been known to prevent heart attacks, and it could reduce your risk of colon cancer, too. Unfortunately, one study found that it takes 10 years of regular aspirin use, four to six tablets a week, to significantly reduce your risk. A recent study done on rats suggests that acetaminophen (Tylenol) could block the cancer-causing substances in foods and help prevent colon cancer, but more studies are needed.

Stop smoking. If the possibility of developing lung cancer frightens you, consider the increased risk of the second-highest cancer killer, too. A recent study found that smokers were more likely to have colon polyps than nonsmokers, and their polyps tended to be more aggressive. The good news from the study was that stopping smoking decreased risk dramatically. Even if you've been smoking most of your life, it's worth the effort to quit. Talk to your doctor about new programs and medications that may help.

Ingredient in your jellies could 'preserve' your life

The stuff that helps turn fruit into jelly might help you lower your risk of colon cancer. This natural, safe and inexpensive product comes from the peel of citrus fruits and apple pulp.

It's called pectin, and it's the fiber that puts the gel in your jellies. And it seems to offer double-barreled protection against both colon cancer and high cholesterol.

Researchers have known for some time that certain parts of fruits and vegetables offer health benefits. In fact, the type of fiber found in fruits and vegetables that is known as "cellulose-derived fiber" helps cut the risk of colon cancer by about 50 percent in laboratory tests.

However, pectin now seems to offer even more health benefits than cellulose-derived fiber. Research shows that rats fed a 10-percent pectin diet experienced the same 50-percent decrease in colon cancer incidence as those fed a diet with cellulose-derived fiber.

However, those on the pectin diet also experienced the additional benefit of a 25- to 30-percent decrease in cholesterol levels. And, lower cholesterol levels help protect you from problems such as high blood pressure and heart disease.

In other words, the cellulose-derived fiber is good for protection against colon cancer alone. In addition, the pectin is good for protection against colon cancer and against high cholesterol.

Scientists think that pectin helps protect against colon cancer by interfering with cancer-causing agents in the colon. And it helps lower cholesterol by preventing the small intestines from absorbing extra fats.

Researchers suggest that in order to achieve the level of protective effects of pectin seen in the research, you would need to eat a lot of fruits and vegetables — even up to 15 apples a day. So, scientists are exploring the possibility of adding pectin to food products to create "pectin-fortified" foods.

Until then, however, even eating a small amount of fruits and vegetables each day will give you some protection. For double-barreled protection against colon cancer and high choles-terol, start with an apple a day, but don't stop there.

Adding more fruits and vegetables to your diet will help give you maximum health benefits.

The easiest way to get enough pectin in your diet might be to add it to your desserts. A couple of teaspoons of powdered fruit pectin, available at some health food stores, can be added to baked goods. Other natural sources of pectin are grapefruit, oranges, sour plums, Concord grapes, gooseberries and vegetables such as carrots and cabbage.

Eating prunes, which contain pectin, also helps lower your cholesterol. In fact, studies report that eating 12 prunes each day can help lower your cholesterol in just four weeks.

Depression

Fish oil — a fat that fights depression

Don't be offended if someone calls you a fathead. You're in good company. Albert Einstein, Thomas Edison, Sir Isaac Newton, and Confucius can be called fatheads, too. That's because fat makes up about 60 percent of the human brain.

But you do have a choice over what type of fathead you want to be. You can keep your brain running smoothly with the right kinds of fats or you can gum up the works with too much of the wrong kind. It all depends on what you eat.

Sound fishy? As a matter of fact, it is. The essential fats found in seafood, called omega-3 fatty acids, play a major role in brain function. They may even boost your mood.

Defeat depression. Next time you're feeling blue, dip into the deep blue sea for your dinner. New medical evidence suggests that the omega-3 fatty acids found in fish — called docosahexaenoic acid (DHA) and eicosapentaenoic acid (EPA) — can help drive away depression.

Dr. Andrew Stoll, a Harvard psychiatrist, found that fish oil capsules helped people with bipolar disorder, or manic depression. People with this condition go through periods of extreme highs and lows. During a high period, they might engage in reckless behavior like spending large sums of money foolishly, while during a low spell they might not get out of bed.

In his study, Dr. Stoll gave fish oil capsules to 14 people with bipolar disorder and a placebo to 16 others. Only 13 percent of the people taking the fish oil capsules experienced any return of depression or mania, compared with 52 percent for the placebo group. And the people taking the fish oil capsules performed significantly better than the placebo group on every test given to measure levels of depression.

According to Dr. Stoll, "The striking difference in relapse rates and response appeared to be highly clinically significant."

Dr. Stoll suggests that the omega-3 fatty acid in the fish oil capsules may act by slowing down neurons in the brain, similar to the drug Lithium, which is used to treat manic depression.

"Although the data are preliminary, our study indicates omega-3 fatty acids are safe and beneficial for patients with bipolar disorder," Dr. Stoll said. "Our finding opens the door for more research on omega-3 fatty acid's effect on a variety of other psychiatric disorders, including major depression, schizophrenia, and attention deficit hyperactivity disorder."

Plenty of other researchers have found links between omega-3 fatty acids and depression. One group from Sheffield, England, noticed that depressed people had much fewer omega-3 fatty acids in their red blood cells than healthy people. The more severe the depression, the less omega-3.

Dr. Joseph Hibbeln of the National Institutes of Health (NIH) in Bethesda, Md., reported similar findings in people across different cultures. For example, in Japan, where annual fish consumption is quite high (over 140 pounds per person), the rate of major depression is only .12 percent. That's a little more than one person with major depression out of every 1,000. On the other hand, in New Zealand, where people eat less than 40 pounds of fish per year, the rate of major depression is 5.8 percent, or 58 per 1,000.

Even though this doesn't prove that eating fish makes you less depressed, the evidence still packs a wallop.

"I am impressed that the two are so closely related," Dr. Hibbeln said. "I was very surprised at the power of the relationship, and I have been impressed that the relationship exists not only for major depression but also appears to exist for other depressive disorders."

There is even evidence that EPA can help treat people with schizophrenia, a serious mental illness that can cause delusions, hallucinations, and disorganized behavior.

Why does fish seem to fight depression? That's a good question without a definite answer. But science provides some strong ideas.

Neurotransmitters, the brain's Pony Express riders that carry messages from cell to cell, have an easier time wriggling through fat membranes made of fluid omega-3 than any other kind of fat. This means your brain's important messages get delivered, not denied access by membranes made of thick, hard fat.

Plus, eating fish has an effect on the levels of serotonin, one of your brain's good-news messengers. People with low levels of serotonin are more likely to be depressed, violent, and suicidal. If you have low levels of DHA, you also have low levels of serotonin. More DHA means more serotonin.

Most antidepressants, including Prozac, raise brain levels of serotonin. You might be doing the same thing just by eating fish. In other words, gills may be as good as pills.

Rethink your ratio. Whether you're depressed or not, chances are you should work more omega-3 into your diet. But it's not as simple as that. You'll probably also have to cut down on omega-6, another type of essential fatty acid found in vegetable oils, meat, milk, and eggs.

Omega-3 and omega-6 are polyunsaturated fatty acids your brain needs but can't make on its own.

"Essential fatty acids only appear through your diet," said Dr. William Lands of the NIH. "What you eat makes you what you are. You can't make 'em. So if you got 'em, it means you ate 'em."

Right now, the typical American eats at least 10 times more omega-6 than omega-3, or a ratio of 10-to-1. Some people's diets push that ratio to 25-to-1 or even higher.

It wasn't always that way. According to Dr. Hibbeln, thousands of years ago ancient people possibly ate five times more omega-3 than omega-6. And who ever heard of a depressed caveman?

But diets changed as people switched from hunting and gathering to an industrial society. They began eating less fruits, vegetables, and fish and more grain and farm-raised meat, not to mention processed foods. It's a menu that put the omega-6 to omega-6 ratio out of whack.

Not that omega-6 is bad. But when one type of fatty acid so outnumbers the other, things can go haywire. Too much omega-6 leads to too much signaling in your brain. With all the hyperactive omega-6 signals running wild, your brain becomes a house full of rowdy teenagers with the parents away for the weekend. This chaos can lead to headaches, arthritis, asthma, arrhythmia, and more. When you take aspirin or ibuprofen, you're getting rid of your headache by cutting down on the excessive omega-6 signaling.

Fortunately, the calmer omega-3 — the parents — can also stop the crazy antics of omega-6 and bring things back to normal. But omega-3 can only do so much in the face of such odds.

Go fish. So, you know why you need to fix your balance of omega-6 and omega-3. But how do you go about doing it?

The obvious first step is to eat more fish. Fatty fish like salmon, herring, mackerel, and tuna offer the most omega-3, but all seafood contains at least some. That's because all fish either eat marine algae, which is rich in the omega-3 fatty acids DHA and EPA, or gobble up other smaller fish that ate the algae.

Aim for at least two fatty fish meals per week. It will also protect your heart. In fact, the American Heart Association recommends two fish meals per week in its dietary guidelines. But if you have heart disease, the suggested number of fish meals per week jumps to seven.

If you're an absolute landlubber who can't stand fish, you can get some omega-3's by eating flaxseed; walnuts; and collard, turnip, and mustard greens. Other good sources include dark green, leafy vegetables like spinach, arugula, kale, Swiss chard, certain types of lettuce, and purslane, a hard-to-find green used in Mediterranean salads.

However, the omega-3 in these foods is in the form of alpha-linolenic acid, which the brain can convert to DHA only in small amounts. So, to get the good stuff your brain prefers, the preformed DHA and EPA, you still need to eat fish. Or you can take fish oil supplements, which are available in health food stores, pharmacies, and supermarkets. (Just one caution — if you're taking blood thinners, you might want to check with your doctor before taking supplements because omega-3 also has a blood-thinning effect.)

"I try to eat at least two to three meals of fish a week, and when I don't eat fish, I try to take supplements," Dr. Hibbeln said.

Just as important are the things he tries not to eat, namely soybean and corn oils, both much too high in omega-6 and too low in omega-3.

"You can do that a number of ways," Dr. Hibbeln said. "One is to completely eliminate all deep-fried foods from your diet. They're bad. Secondly, is to try to eliminate margarine and salad dressings that have corn or soybean oil in them."

Grams of fatty acid per 100 grams (about 1/2 cup or 3 1/2 ounces) of food

Food	Omega-6 fatty acids	Omega-3 fatty acids ALA	EPA	DHA
Beans and legumes				
Lentils, dry	0.4	0.16	–	–
Lima beans, dry	0.5	0.2	–	–
Navy beans, dry	0.2	0.3	–	–
Pinto beans, cooked	0.2	0.3	–	–
Soybeans, cooked	0.4	2.1	–	–
Dairy and fats				
Butter	1.8	1.2	–	–
Cheese, cheddar	0.5	0.4	–	–
Cream, whipping	0.9	0.5	–	–
Egg, yolk	4.2	0.1	–	–
Margarine, hard, soybean	19.4	1.5	–	–
Mayonnaise, soybean	37.1	4.2	–	–
Milk, whole	–	0.1	–	–
Salad dressing, commercial, Italian	24.7	3.3	–	–
Fish and seafood				
Anchovy	0.2	–	0.5	0.9
Bluefish	0.4	–	0.4	0.8
Carp	0.8	0.3	.02	.01
Cod, Atlantic	Trace	Trace	0.1	.02
Crab, Alaska king	–	Trace	0.2	0.1
Flounder	0.1	Trace	0.1	0.1
Halibut, Pacific	0.2	0.1	0.1	0.3
Herring, Pacific	0.6	0.1	1.0	0.7
Mackerel, Atlantic	1.1	0.1	0.9	1.6
Salmon, Atlantic	0.7	0.2	0.3	0.9
Scallop, sea	0.6	0.3	21.3	26.2
Shrimp	0.2	Trace	0.2	0.1
Sole, lemon	0.7	2.0	14.7	6.8
Tuna, albacore	0.3	0.2	0.3	1.0
Fruit				
Avocados, California, raw	1.9	0.1	–	–
Raspberries	0.2	.01	–	–

Food	Omega-6 fatty acids	Omega-3 fatty acids		
		ALA	EPA	DHA
Grain				
Barley, bran	2.4	0.3	–	–
Oats, germ	11.0	1.4	–	–
Rice, bran	6.4	0.2	–	–
Wheat, bran	2.2	0.2	–	–
Wheat, germ	5.9	0.7	–	–
Meat and poultry				
Beef, ground, raw	0.8	0.2	–	–
Beef, T-bone steak, lean, raw	0.3	Trace	–	–
Chicken, light meat	0.4	Trace	Trace	0.02
Nuts and seeds				
Cashews	7.3	0.2	0	0
Flaxseed	7	17	0	0
Peanut	14.4	0.6	0	0
Walnuts, black	34.2	3.3	–	–
Oils				
Canola (rapeseed)	22.2	11.2	–	–
Cod liver	6.6	0.7	9.0	9.5
Flaxseed (linseed)	15	55	0	0
Olive	9	0.7	0	0
Peanut	29	1.1	0	0
Safflower	77	1	–	–
Soybean	53	7	0	0
Walnut	52.9	10.4	–	–
Wheat germ	54.8	6.9	–	–
Vegetables				
Broccoli, raw	0.03	0.1	–	–
Cauliflower, raw	–	0.1	–	–
Corn, germ	17.7	0.3	–	–
Kale, raw	0.1	0.2	–	–
Lettuce, Butterhead, raw	–	0.1	–	–
Mustard	–	0.04	–	–
Purslane	0.09	0.4	–	–
Seaweed, Spirulina, dried	1.2	0.8	–	–
Spinach, raw	0.1	0.9	–	–

Switching from corn or soybean oil to canola oil, which has a more favorable 2-to-1 ratio of omega-6 to omega-3, or to olive oil, a monounsaturated oil with the least amount of omega-6, would do wonders for your essential fatty acid balance.

"Just by throwing away that bottle and putting a new bottle in the kitchen, it makes a big difference."

The same advice — eat more fatty fish, substitute olive or canola oil for other vegetable oils, reduce deep-fried foods — appears in the book *The Omega Diet* by Dr. Artemis P. Simopoulos.

Her book includes recipes and tips for balancing your omega-6 to omega-3 ratio as well as sample three-week menus for breakfast, lunch, and dinner. What jumps out is just how much variety there is in a healthy, balanced diet.

That's also one of the points Dr. Lands has been trying to stress. "On a given day, you can really pig out on something," he said. "But with 30-some days in a month, you've got the rest of the month to atone for a given day's imbalance. Your body will integrate these things over time."

So know what you're eating, because it all boils down to this — what type of fat you eat determines how your brain works. Moreover, your food determines your mood. Just by getting more omega-3 and less omega-6 into your diet, you can put your brain, and your spirits, in high gear.

And that's no fish story.

• •

Boost omega-3s with free computer program

If you want to improve your omega-3 to omega-6 ratio, try using an interactive computer software program called KIM (Keep

It Managed). If you have a personal computer, you can download KIM for free from the NIH's Eicosanoids Web page at <http://intra-mural.niaaa.nih.gov/eicosanoids>.

With KIM, you enter your height, weight, and exercise pattern (very light, moderate, etc.), and KIM gives you a sample menu with a wide range of foods. You can browse through a list of foods and make changes to the menu to improve your omega-3 to omega-6 ratio. It's interesting to see how one change in the menu — for example, substituting tuna for pork at lunch — can significantly lower the ratio.

• •

6 drug-free ways to beat depression

It's a fact of life. Most people get depressed every once in a while. The good news is a long-term study has revealed new ways to treat depression without dangerous drugs.

Enjoy family and friends. Don't just count the number of family members and friends you have — really connect with them. People who are depressed tend to isolate themselves. Stay in touch with your friends and the people you love.

Find meaning in your life. A study conducted by the Northern Arizona University Department of Nursing found that seniors living in retirement communities were less depressed if they had a feeling of purpose and importance that went beyond themselves. A great way to start is by reaching out and helping other people. And learning to appreciate all of the good things in your life is another way to lift your spirits.

Work on staying healthy. People who feel good are less depressed. You'll feel better if you eat well-balanced, healthy meals; get enough sleep; and exercise every day.

Most kinds of physical activity reduce stress, get you out of the house, raise your energy level, encourage you to interact with others, and get your mind off your problems.

Numerous studies show that people participating in regular exercise are less likely to become depressed than people who don't. Exercise actually stimulates the production of dopamine and serotonin, chemicals in your brain that improve your mood. In fact, for some people, it is just as effective as taking antidepressants and getting counseling. In almost all cases, when people add an exercise program to their drug or counseling treatment, their conditions improve more rapidly and significantly.

Your doctor may even prescribe exercise instead of antidepressants. Although the drugs will often bring about a more immediate improvement, in the long run, working out is just as powerful.

Wake up to the light. Depression can affect your sleep. Perhaps you're sleeping too much, or you can't sleep at all. Maybe you wake up several times during the night. When you're tired and have no energy, you feel even more depressed.

These symptoms could mean your internal clock is not running as smoothly as it should. When you adjust your body clock, you adjust your mood. It's easy to do. Simply control the amount and quality of sleep you get each night and how much light you are exposed to at different times of the day.

Even normal levels of indoor, artificial lighting can affect your internal clock. In the evening, dim the lights before winding down. Make your bedroom dark while you sleep. Change your sleep pattern so you are awake in the morning and exposed to as much early daylight as possible. Open your curtains or blinds. Morning sunshine increases the level of melatonin in your body, a hormone that helps regulate your sleep cycle naturally.

You will sleep better at night and wake up feeling more rested and less depressed if you soak up bright light for several hours every day. But don't use ultraviolet (UV) light because experts aren't sure of its safety. The brighter the light and the longer you are exposed, the more helpful it is in treating depression.

Use your sense of smell. Aromatherapy can help treat many physical and emotional problems, from headaches to depression. Researchers have found that vapors in essential oils trigger a specific part of your brain to release chemicals, such as serotonin, into your nervous system. These brain chemicals help relieve depression by calming you or helping you sleep. Many hospitals are using aromatherapy to reduce stress and encourage good sleep patterns in their patients.

Lavender is one of the most well-known and versatile herbs. In a study at the University of Miami School of Medicine, researchers found that just three minutes of aromatherapy with a lavender scent were not only relaxing but relieved depression, too.

To fight the blues, surround yourself with juniper, marjoram, melissa, or orange blossom. Add them to your bath; massage with them; use a diffuser, vaporizer, candles, aroma lamps, or potpourri burners; spray them in the air; or inhale them straight from the bottle.

Find healing with herbs. In a study of about 300 people, St. John's wort was just as effective as one of the leading antidepressants in improving quality of life, both emotionally and physically. This is great news because herbal supplements have fewer and less severe side effects than most antidepressants. That means people are more likely to continue taking the supplement.

St. John's wort is a good, safe choice for mild to moderate depression but not severe depression, manic-depression, or obsessive-compulsive disorder.

Other herbs used to treat depression are kava and valerian. But remember — since herbal supplements are not regulated, even similar products can vary greatly.

If you want to use herbs to treat your depression, ask your doctor for advice. Don't stop taking any medicine without his approval, and continue seeing him regularly so he can monitor your depression.

Lift your spirits with good nutrition

Would life seem better if you had a pint of chocolate ice cream in front of you? Certain foods can boost or suppress the amount of chemicals in your brain. Some of these chemicals, like serotonin, help make you happier, calmer, energetic, alert, and more relaxed.

Don't ignore the connection between your mood and your diet. If you want to chase away the blues, experts say, look at what's on your plate.

Begin with breakfast. People who always start their day with a cereal-rich breakfast may be less stressed and less depressed than those who eat breakfast only now and then — at least that's what researchers say. And if you regularly eat breakfast, you are more likely to be in good health, be a nonsmoker, and drink less alcohol — all factors that can contribute to a better frame of mind.

Eat more grains, fruits, and veggies. Experts say complex carbohydrates, found in vegetables, fruits, and grains like oats, can trigger the production of serotonin. Raising the level of serotonin in your brain can help raise your spirits.

Pick up some protein. Researchers have found a direct link between depression and low levels of protein in the diet. In one study, not only did depression increase as people stuck to a low-protein diet, but their lifestyle and quality of life also declined.

Most people get more than enough protein, but if you don't, add a little meat and dairy products to your diet.

Hook a few fish. Omega-3 fatty acids, found in fish that live in cold, deep water, may also help you win the battle against depression. In countries where people eat a lot of salmon, sardines, mackerel, herring, anchovies, and tuna, the incidence of depression is low. If you have a richer taste, caviar is also high in omega-3. Experts say the omega-3 fatty acids in fish oil may suppress certain overactive brain signals. Eat fatty fish three or four times a week to get enough of this important nutrient.

If you have manic depression, talk with your doctor about fish oil supplements. Researchers at Harvard Medical School and Baylor College of Medicine say taking fish oil supplements daily can help control the extreme mood swings that come with manic depression.

Keep your caffeine routine. If you don't feel like yourself until after your first cup of coffee, you're not alone. Many people say caffeine keeps them alert and improves their mood. Now medical evidence is starting to back this up. In a 10-year study of female nurses, caffeine seemed to make a big difference in the rate of serious depression. Women who were regular coffee drinkers had lower rates of suicide than women who didn't drink coffee. While you shouldn't deal with depression by drinking four pots of coffee every morning, how much or how little caffeine you consume could be affecting the way you look at the world.

Lose weight slowly. If you are a woman who has ever suffered from major depression, going on a diet may increase your chances of another run-in with this frustrating illness. In clinical tests, a regimen of about 1,000 calories a day didn't supply enough tryptophan, a chemical needed to produce the brain chemical serotonin. Women who had never experienced depression before automatically adjusted to the low serotonin levels. The women who had a history of depression did not adjust and became very depressed.

This doesn't mean if you go on a diet you are going to become depressed. It does mean, however, that you should choose a weight loss program carefully and talk with your doctor if you notice any changes in your mood.

Forgo the fat. You've been warned against the dangers of too much fat for years — it clogs your arteries, balloons your hips, and it may be bad for your brain, too.

Studies find that people with a high level of triglycerides in their blood are more likely to suffer from mental problems, like depression. In one study, researchers put people who were depressed on a low-fat diet for 54 weeks and gave them medication to help lower their triglycerides. As their triglyceride level fell, their depression was relieved. At the end of the study, 91 percent of the people were back to normal.

Boost your brain with B vitamins. Folic acid is an important B vitamin that helps maintain serotonin levels in your brain. Without enough folic acid, you could experience depression or other mental disorders. Good sources of folic acid include liver; beans; and green, leafy vegetables, like spinach.

A deficiency of vitamin B6 interferes with your brain's ability to make neurotransmitters and can lead to depression, shortened attention span, and other mental problems. Potatoes, bananas, and chicken are rich in vitamin B6.

An estimated 80 to 90 percent of people with a vitamin B12 deficiency will develop some sort of nervous system disorder. This vitamin helps your body manufacture the neurotransmitters that prevent memory loss, depression, and other mood disorders. B12 is only found in foods from animal origins, so strict vegetarians may need to take supplements. Beef, dairy products, and fish are good sources of vitamin B12.

Uncover hidden causes of depression

One out of every 10 Americans suffers a serious bout of depression at some point in his life. If you are depressed, talk with your doctor. It's possible your depression might be caused by one of these health problems.

Hypothyroidism. If you have a bad case of the blues, get your thyroid checked. It might not be producing enough thyroxine, a hormone that affects metabolism. Too little can make you feel depressed and slow, both physically and mentally — and antidepressants won't help.

High or low testosterone. In men, high or low testosterone levels can cause depression. If you have either too much or too little, you are at greater risk of depression. Ask your doctor to check your testosterone level.

Diabetes. The American Diabetes Association says people with diabetes are more likely to suffer from depression than the rest of the population. Although one does not necessarily cause the other, they are likely to be related. Get professional help since both conditions, diabetes and depression, need to be medically treated.

Stroke. In some cases, small clots in your brain's blood vessels can cause depression. These lesions can form after a "silent stroke" — an episode that has no outward symptoms but still damages the brain. Silent strokes interfere with the way your brain functions, possibly triggering depression. These strokes are warnings that you are at risk of experiencing a major stroke.

Low cholesterol. It's a controversial idea — very low cholesterol can cause depression. Organizations like the American Heart Association and the Food and Drug Administration are not convinced, but several respected researchers say it's true.

A Duke University study found that very low levels of LDL cholesterol, the kind associated with heart disease, and triglycerides went hand-in-hand with depression and anxiety in otherwise healthy, middle-age women. It was the same for younger women tested by the Swedish Department of Public Health Sciences. Regardless of other health factors, like weight and exercise, if their cholesterol was low, the women were more likely to be depressed or anxious. Researchers say this connection may only occur in people with naturally low cholesterol, not in people who lower high levels through diet and exercise.

Skeptics feel there could be other factors causing the depression. Many are hesitant to advise people against lowering their cholesterol because of the increased risk of heart disease.

Know your cholesterol levels — very low levels fall below 160 milligrams (mg) per deciliter. If your cholesterol is low and you are depressed, talk with your doctor.

Diabetes

5 natural ways to beat diabetes

The best way to control your diabetes is to become more active in managing the disease. Talk with your doctor about an exercise and diet plan, and then ask about these natural remedies that just might make life a little easier.

Cornstarch. Cornstarch does more than just thicken your gravy. It's a starch that's digested and absorbed slowly, so it helps maintain a stable amount of glucose in your bloodstream over a period of time.

It can also head off trouble if you have insulin-dependent (type I) diabetes. Type I diabetics are particularly prone to low blood glucose levels overnight. Researchers discovered that uncooked cornstarch dissolved in a nonsugary drink, such as milk or sugar-free soda, helped control diabetics' blood glucose levels overnight. But remember — before trying this remedy, talk with your doctor.

Look for new snack bars that contain sucrose, protein, and uncooked cornstarch. These three ingredients release glucose at different speeds, giving you both immediate and long-term help for hypoglycemia, or low blood sugar.

Hot tubs. You may think there's nothing more relaxing than soaking in a hot tub, but did you ever think it could help your diabetes? Some experts say it improves blood flow to your muscles, just like exercise. This could be especially important to diabetics who are unable to exercise. In one study, diabetics who soaked for a half-hour each day, six days a week, for three weeks, lost weight, lowered their average blood glucose level, slept better, and generally felt healthier. One participant was even able to reduce his insulin by 18 percent.

Before you take the plunge, here are some things to watch out for.

- If the water is very hot and you stand up quickly or exit the hot tub in a hurry, you may become dizzy. This can be dangerous if you're not holding onto a handrail for support.

- If you've lost feeling in your feet due to diabetic neuropathy, make sure the water isn't so hot it can burn your skin.

- Monitor the chemicals in your hot tub. They are there to kill harmful bacteria. Soaking in hot water can leave your skin vulnerable to injury and infection.

Capsaicin cream. If diabetes has left you suffering from troublesome skin pain, try this natural remedy — capsaicin skin cream. It's made from the same red peppers you use to spice up your chili. When applied to your skin, it is absorbed and gradually deadens nerves that transmit pain. It may take two to four weeks to bring on any noticeable changes, but hang in there. It's a natural, safe alternative that's proved effective for several painful conditions, including arthritis and shingles. Look for capsaicin products in cream or lotion form. They are available over-the-counter or by prescription.

Chromium. Insulin is the hormone that moves glucose, or sugar, out of your bloodstream and into your cells. Chromium is the mineral that helps insulin do its work. Several studies prove chromium supplements help diabetics lower their blood sugar and improve their insulin levels. And taking chromium dramatically improved the severe shaking, blurred vision, sleepiness, and heavy sweating for a group of people with hypoglycemia. If more research confirms these numbers, experts say chromium supplements may become standard treatment for diabetes.

There's no Recommended Dietary Allowance (RDA) for chromium, but the Estimated Safe and Adequate Daily Dietary Intake for healthy adults is 50 to 200 micrograms (mcg) per day. In several clinical studies, diabetics took 600 to 1,000 mcg per day. Don't take this much without talking with your doctor first. To get more chromium naturally, eat asparagus, beef, brewer's yeast, calves' liver, chicken, dairy products, eggs, fish and seafood, mushrooms, nuts, potatoes with skin, prunes, whole-grain products, and fresh fruit, especially apples with skin.

Milk thistle. *Silybum marianum*, also known as silymarin, is an herb whose seeds, fruit, and leaves have been used for food and medicine for over 2,000 years. Although a popular treatment for liver disorders, early research indicates milk thistle may be helpful for diabetics. It seems to lower glucose levels without causing hypoglycemia. This may help in preventing and treating diabetic complications. Even though several herbal experts support using milk thistle for liver problems, the research is still too new for diabetes. Talk with your doctor about this natural treatment and be on the lookout for more news.

●●●●●●●●●●●●●●●●●●●●●●●●●●●●●
Emergency treatment for low blood sugar

If you are shaking, sweating, and feeling weak, you may be suffering from hypoglycemia or low blood sugar. The best treatment is to eat something, preferably something containing sugar, and you should feel better in about 15 minutes.

These suggestions come from *U.S. Pharmacist*:

- a piece of fruit

- 1/4 to 1/3 cup of raisins

- 1/2 cup fruit juice

- eight Lifesavers

- 4 to 6 ounces of a sugared soft drink

- 2 or 3 (5-gram) glucose tablets

- one tube of glucose gel

- 1 cup skim milk

• • • • • • • • • • • • • • • • • • • •

Instant help from a tiny seed

If you have type II diabetes, also known as noninsulin de-pendent diabetes mellitus (NIDDM), there's a simple step you can take at mealtimes to lower your blood sugar and help keep your diabetes under control. The secret is a water-soluble fiber from the psyllium seed.

Psyllium seed husk is technically an herb. It acts as both an over-the-counter drug, in products like Metamucil and other bulk laxatives, and as a food additive in many breakfast cereals, like Kellogg's Bran Buds.

As early as 1985, research showed psyllium helped control blood sugar levels. Now new studies confirm that psyllium is especially effective against NIDDM.

In separate trials, psyllium before meals caused blood glucose levels to drop from 9 to 20 percent in people with NIDDM. And it doesn't seem to matter if you're already taking drugs to lower your blood sugar or if you're trying to control it with diet alone. The results are just as amazing.

The amounts tested varied, but most experts recommend only 5 grams (or about one teaspoon) with water, three times a day, before meals. It's an easy thing to do at home or on the go. There are usually no side effects as long as you drink plenty of water each day and don't go over the recommended amount. That's because too much fiber can cause diarrhea and bloating. An added bonus — including psyllium in your regular diet will help lower your cholesterol level, too.

●●●●●●●●●●●●●●●●●●●●●●●●●●●

New no-pain ways to check glucose

Tired of constantly pricking your finger to check blood glucose levels? If you have diabetes, you may think this is just a fact of life. Well, not anymore.

Researchers have come up with two new ways to check your insulin levels without shedding a single drop of blood. Painless testing methods like these will improve the quality of life for millions of people with diabetes.

GlucoWatch. Strap the GlucoWatch onto your wrist, and you'll receive blood glucose readings through your skin three times an hour — all without doing a thing. Using a continuous, low-level electric current, this device compares each reading to an earlier one, actually providing more information about glucose levels than other methods. It's accurate, painless, automatic, hardly noticeable, and can go anywhere. You can also set an alarm to sound whenever glucose levels drop too low, preventing dangerous hypoglycemia attacks. The device will cost around $300, and it should last two to three years. If you're over 18, talk with your doctor about the GlucoWatch. It has received preliminary FDA approval and should be available soon.

Ultrasound. Doctors use ultrasound today for a lot more than looking at babies. It can reduce inflammation in injured muscles, clean teeth, and even monitor your blood glucose. A two-minute burst of ultrasound on the back of your forearm allows the glucose to cross through your skin where it can be measured for up to 12 hours. Researchers are developing a hand-held device that you'll be able to use at home.

●●●●●●●●●●●●●●●●●●●●●●●

Coping with driving and hypoglycemia

Have you ever felt dizzy, uncoordinated, shaky, and sweaty? If you have diabetes, you know these are symptoms of hypoglycemia — your blood sugar is too low. When this happens, resting for a minute and having a snack can help. But what happens if you're behind the wheel?

Research shows you may not always make the best decisions about your condition and your ability to drive safely. If you get behind the wheel, you can pose a safety risk to yourself and others.

Scientists, using hand-held computers, asked diabetics to estimate their blood sugar levels. Next, they measured their actual blood sugar levels, tested basic math skills, and gauged reaction times. About 60 percent of the time, the diabetics said they would drive even though their blood sugar levels tested low enough to impair their driving ability.

Learn to pay attention to the signs that indicate your blood sugar is too high or too low. Measure your blood glucose level before driving. Know when low is too low. And carry sugary snacks with you for emergencies.

● ●
Are you an 'apple' or a 'pear'?

You've probably heard that it's better to be a "pear." Pear-shaped people carry their extra weight in their hips and thighs and are less likely to develop heart disease than apple-shaped people, who carry their extra weight in their abdomens.

Now a new study has uncovered more bad news for "apples" — or at least for apple-shaped women. The study found that women who tended to store body fat in their abdominal area were more likely to be insulin resistant — and, therefore, more likely to develop diabetes.

If you don't have that desirable, perfect pear shape, don't panic. It just means you need to be aware of your increased risk and work extra hard to keep that fat away from your tummy.

• •

Another reason to take a walk

Worried about developing diabetes? If so, take comfort in knowing there is something you can do to cut your risk in half — take a walk. You don't have to run marathons or be physically active in your job. Just spend your free time getting up off the couch.

Researchers found that brisk walking is as healthful as more vigorous forms of exercise. This is good news since walking is something almost everyone can do. It's cheap, rarely causes injury, can be done almost anywhere, and you don't have to be in great shape to start.

What's important is how much energy you use. Think about tasks you do in and around your home every day. If you push a lawn mower, scrub the floor, or even run laundry up and down the stairs, you are helping your body fight this serious disease. Both the Centers for Disease Control and Prevention and the National Institutes of Health recommend getting at least 30 minutes of fairly vigorous exercise every day.

An 8-year study found that exercise was more important in determining diabetes risk than diet, weight, or heredity. Exercise helps control your weight, which lowers your risk for diabetes, but it may also help your body process glucose.

And remember, it's never too early or too late to get started. Statistics show if you are overweight when you are 25, you are more likely to be diabetic in middle age. That doesn't mean give up on your health if you're over 40. It just means everyone, young and old, needs to add exercise to their daily routines.

Diarrhea

Relief for diarrhea

What you choose to eat when you have diarrhea can make a big difference in your recovery — so choose carefully.

Cook up some rice. Want a simple, safe, yet inexpensive treatment? Boil some rice. Scientists have discovered a substance in cooked rice that keeps your intestinal cells from producing too much chloride, which can cause diarrhea. Many underdeveloped countries have been using this remedy for years. They simply drink the cooled water left in the pot after cooking rice. In addition to inhibiting your chloride secretion, this liquid contains starch and nutrients that help rehydrate and restore your system.

Bite into an apple. This juicy fruit can relieve both diarrhea *and* constipation. Apples contain pectin, a soluble fiber, that absorbs water in your stomach and intestines. It swells and forms a gummy mass that moistens and softens the stool to help ease difficult bowel movements. At the same time, the bulk formed by pectin firms up the watery stool of diarrhea, changing it to a thicker consistency.

Drink plenty of liquids. When you have diarrhea, you lose body fluids. It's important to replace the lost water and electrolytes — salts and minerals normally found in your blood, tissue fluids, and cells. Drink at least eight to 10 glasses of liquid each day to replenish your body's fluids. Water, caffeine-free sodas, popsicles, herbal tea, broth, or gelatin are good choices. Or try this recipe — mix one teaspoon of salt and four teaspoons of sugar into one quart of water. Drink two cups of this every hour.

Eat some berries. Dried blueberries are a popular European remedy for diarrhea. If you can't find them at your grocery store, make your own. Simply spread some fresh berries out in the sun until they wrinkle and shrivel up. Then, either eat about three tablespoons of the berries or crush them, boil them for 10 minutes, strain, and drink as a tea. Remember — eating fresh blueberries won't have the same effect. Another choice is the bilberry. It's a variety of blueberry that also works well on diarrhea. You may find dried bilberries or bilberry extract in your local herb shop.

Give the BRAT a try. To ease your digestive system back onto solids after a bout with diarrhea, try the BRAT diet. Instead of moving right from water to normal eating, the BRAT method suggests a transitional diet of Bananas, Rice, Applesauce, and Toast. These foods are both nutritious and gentle on your digestive tract. After things have returned to normal, eat soft, bland foods, such as cooked cereal, rice, eggs, custard, bananas, yogurt, soda crackers, toast, skinless baked potatoes, or chicken for a while longer.

Beware of these grains. Are you suffering from diarrhea after a particular meal? Think about what you just ate. If your menu included wheat, rye, barley, or another grain, you may be allergic to gluten, a mixture of proteins found in these grains. This inherited allergy, called celiac sprue disease, can severely damage the lining of your intestines. If you think this may be causing your problems, try substituting products made with rice, corn, or soybean flour.

Take it slowly. For several days after experiencing diarrhea, stay away from fruit; alcohol; caffeine; milk; gassy foods, like beans, cabbage, and onions; and spicy, greasy, or fatty foods.

• •
Say 'No way!' to traveler's diarrhea

If you eat food or drink water contaminated with bacteria, like *E. coli,* you're likely to get a bad case of diarrhea, nausea, and vomiting. It's not usually life-threatening, but it can certainly be uncomfortable.

Although you can be infected with these bacteria almost anywhere, less-developed countries without modern sewage and water treatment facilities are especially risky. In fact, the illness is so common in popular vacation destinations like Mexico and Central and South America, that it's known as traveler's diarrhea.

If you don't want to be the next victim of Montezuma's revenge, practice these travel tips:

- Don't use tap water for drinking or brushing your teeth. Buy bottled water.

- Before eating, clean your hands with packaged wipes or antiseptic cleanser, not tap water.

- Drink bottled water, boiled coffee or tea, carbonated drinks, beer, or wine only.

- Order your drinks without ice.

- Eat fruits, like bananas, you can peel yourself.

- Don't eat raw vegetables or salads. Eat thoroughly cooked, hot food.

- Buy food and drinks from reputable restaurants and hotels, not street vendors.

- Pack some bromelain, a pineapple enzyme that may block *E. coli.*

• •

Nicotine patch cancels out colitis

If you suffer from diarrhea and abdominal cramps as a result of colitis, a nicotine patch may provide relief.

Several studies have found that the nicotine patch and nicotine gum may ease symptoms of colitis. This condition affects about half a million people in the United States.

In the latest study, people with colitis who hadn't found relief from conventional drug treatment were given a nicotine patch or a look-alike patch without nicotine. The people who wore the nicotine patches were four times more likely to experience an improvement in symptoms than the people who wore the other patches.

If you have colitis, and medication hasn't helped, talk to your doctor about trying the patch. Nicotine patches can cause side effects, and some people shouldn't use them.

Drug side effects

10 tips to prevent dangerous medical mistakes

Improved medical care and new medications have enabled people to live longer, but sometimes they can cause problems or even death.

According to a report by the Institute of Medicine, as many as 44,000 to 98,000 people in the United States die in hospitals each year as the result of medical errors. Another study found that side effects from medications may be more common than previously thought because many people don't report adverse reactions to their doctors.

Everybody makes mistakes, including doctors and nurses. That's why you have to look out for your own health by being an active participant in your medical care.

Be a wise consumer. About 75 percent of doctors' appointments end with at least one prescription being written. Make sure you get the most out of your medicine by following these suggestions.

- Tell your doctor about any other medications you are taking. This includes over-the-counter medications, like pain relievers and sleeping pills, as well as herbs or other supplements.

- Tell your doctor about any side effects or allergic reactions you've had to medications in the past. Often, drugs that are related will cause the same sort of reaction.

- Ask about side effects. Being aware of a drug's side effects can help you determine if a problem is caused by your medication or by another medical condition.

- Make sure you understand your prescription. Doctors are notorious for having bad handwriting, so make sure you know what the prescription is for. If you can't read it, your pharmacist may not be able to, either. It's a good idea to write down the name of the medicine, as well as dosage information, in your own handwriting.

- Compare the medicine label to your prescription. One study found that 88 percent of prescription errors involved the wrong drug or the wrong dose. When you pick up your prescription, compare the name and instructions on the label to the ones on your prescription.

- Ask questions. If there's anything you don't understand about your prescription, don't hesitate to ask your doctor or pharmacist.

Have a safe hospital stay. Most people will have at least one hospital stay in their lifetimes. Make sure yours is a safe one.

- Choose the right hospital. If you have a choice, ask how many people with your condition are treated at each hospital you are considering. Research shows that you are more likely to have a successful visit if you choose a hospital with more experience in treating your condition or doing the particular procedure or surgery you need.

- Ask about handwashing. The spread of infection from patient to patient can be a problem in hospitals, and handwashing is an important step in preventing it. Don't be afraid to ask anyone responsible for your care if they've washed their hands.

- If you're having surgery, make sure you and the surgeon are in agreement on what you're having done — and where. While surgical mistakes like operating on the wrong site (for example, the left knee instead of the right) are rare, taking a few moments to confirm a procedure with your surgeon could avert a disaster. The American Academy of Orthopaedic Surgeons recommends that surgeons sign their initials directly on the site to be operated on before the surgery.

• Ask questions — again and again! Make sure you know what is being done to you and why. And when it's time to leave the hospital, make sure you understand what kind of follow-up care you're supposed to have.

Choosing wisely — brand names or generics?

When you get a prescription filled, the pharmacist will often ask if you want a generic substitute. You know generics are less expensive, but you may not be sure if the quality is the same as the name-brand medicine you are used to. After all, you get what you pay for, right?

While buying brand-name items might be worth the extra money for some products, when it comes to medicine, the quality should be exactly the same. Generic drugs have to pass the same standards set by the Food and Drug Administration (FDA) as brand name drugs. So why the big price difference?

Research and development for a new drug can take years, and millions of dollars. That's why the government allows a company that develops a new drug at least 10 years patent protection. During that time, no other company can copy the drug. This means the company can make back the money it spent developing the drug. Doing this encourages companies to continue developing new drugs.

When the 10-year patent protection period ends, companies that manufacture generic drugs are free to copy the formula. The

FDA requires that generic drugs be equivalent to the brand name drug it is copying. The only difference is that manufacturers of a generic drug are allowed to use different inactive ingredients and fillers. This is why the generic drug may not look the same as the name brand.

If you're still unsure about whether to buy generic, talk to your doctor or pharmacist.

Ear problems

An action plan for healthy ears

The delicate mechanisms that make up your inner ear are very sensitive. You can damage your hearing doing ordinary, everyday things without even realizing you are doing any harm. To keep your ears healthy, try these tips:

Turn down the volume. Whether it's a firecracker on the Fourth of July or the tools in your woodworking shop, there are two ways you can lose your hearing — suddenly from a single, strong noise or gradually from being continually exposed to high-level noise. To prevent this from happening to you, recognize which noises are in the danger zone and wear ear plugs or protective headphones when you're around them.

0 decibels	threshold of normal hearing
20 decibels	whispered voice
40 decibels	refrigerator humming
60 decibels	normal conversation
80 decibels	city traffic
90 decibels	lawn mower, motorcycle
100 decibels	woodworking shop
110 decibels	chainsaw
120 decibels	boom cars, snowmobile
140 decibels	rock concerts, firecrackers

If you are exposed to any noise over 90 decibels for a long period of time, you may experience gradual hearing loss. At 100 decibels, just 15 minutes without earplugs can cause ear damage. And listening to 110 decibels for more than a minute can cause permanent hearing loss.

Exercise regularly. Add hearing to the list of things exercise helps. Exercise improves the circulation of blood to your inner ear where it helps keep hearing mechanisms, such as your sound-detecting hair cells, in good working order.

Don't strain. Extreme physical stress can raise the level of pressure in your ears to a dangerous level and cause damage to your hearing. Use extra caution when lifting heavy objects or exerting yourself in any way.

Play it safe with pets. Do you love animals? Do your animals love you? If they show it by licking your ears, this little sign of affection could quickly turn into infection. Many pets, including dogs and cats, can pass bacteria in their saliva to humans. And if your pet licks your ear, this bacteria can easily infect the delicate structures inside your ear canals. This means big trouble, especially if you have a perforated eardrum or a history of ear problems. So go ahead and love Fido, but give up the doggie kisses and settle for a handshake.

Keep your ears dry. Whether you swim laps every day, enjoy a water aerobics class, or simply jump in and out of the shower, your ears get wet. And wet ears are the perfect breeding ground for bacteria and fungus. This combination often results in an outer ear infection called swimmer's ear. You can buy remedies at almost any drugstore, but here's a quick and cheap way to make your own. Mix equal parts of isopropyl rubbing alcohol and white vinegar in a small bottle. The alcohol dries out the moisture, and the vinegar discourages the growth of bacteria and fungus. Apply a few drops in each ear.

Chew some gum. Chewing the right kind of gum may end ear infections forever. A natural sweetener called xylitol prevents bacteria from attaching itself to the back of your mouth, where it can later enter your ear and set off an infection. One study of preschool children found that chewing gum with xylitol cut the incidence of ear infection in half.

Get professional help. You need to see a specialist if you answer "yes" to three or more of the following questions:

- Do you have a problem hearing over the telephone?

- Do you have trouble following the conversation when two or more people are talking at the same time?

- Do people complain that you turn the TV volume up too high?

- Do you have to strain to understand conversation?

- Do you have trouble hearing in a noisy background?

- Do you find yourself asking people to repeat themselves?

- Do many people you talk to seem to mumble (or not speak clearly)?

- Do you misunderstand what others are saying and respond inappropriately?

- Do you have trouble understanding the speech of women and children?

- Do people get annoyed because you misunderstand what they say?

For a quick, free test of your hearing, call Dial a Hearing Test at 1-800-222-EARS (3277). They'll give you a local number you can call to take a two-minute hearing test over the phone.

● ●
Check your medicine

Some drugs can cause or contribute to hearing loss. Aspirin, furosemide, neomycin, and gentamicin are common culprits. If you take any of these drugs, have your hearing checked regularly.

● ●

Earwax: What it is and what to do about it

Most people don't understand the purpose of earwax and consider it to be something dirty that has to be cleaned out. Others feel that wax buildup causes infections. But, according to researchers, earwax has gotten a bad rap over the years.

Earwax is a friend, not a foe. Earwax is a natural product that your body makes to help keep foreign particles from getting to and damaging your fragile eardrum. It protects your ears from infection. It traps dust, sand, insects and other particles and keeps them from getting into the ears.

In most cases, earwax gets rid of itself by traveling outward, drying up and flaking away. Unfortunately, many people have earwax-producing cells in their ear canals that work overtime. You end up with too much wax.

Apparently, you can run into some problems when you attempt to clean your ears out yourself. The softer wax can get pushed back into the ear, block the canal and get trapped. The wax can become impacted and then you've got trouble.

Other reasons why wax can become impacted in your ears are an increase in the number of hairs in your ears as you age, producing an unusual amount of wax, or abnormally shaped ear canals. Lack of chewing your food properly can also keep the wax from migrating out.

Devices that fit into the ears such as hearing aids, stethoscopes or molded earpieces can also create problems leading to excessive earwax.

Too much wax in your ears can cause hearing problems, ringing in the ear and just simple problems with personal hygiene. Symptoms of wax buildup can range from slight annoyance to severe pain in the ear. It can sometimes cause hearing loss, dizziness and vertigo.

Australian researchers tested several commonly used products for ear wax removal and found that the best one just happens to be the cheapest — sodium bicarbonate. Just mix one teaspoon of sodium bicarbonate in two teaspoons of water. Shake well and apply a few drops in your ear with a dropper. Within one hour, the solution should break up the wax. Although oil, the most commonly used remedy, won't dissolve ear wax away, the researchers admit it might lubricate your ear canal enough so you can remove the wax easily — but it's much messier.

Most drug stores or pharmacies sell over-the-counter ear cleansing kits. The kits include some eardrops that will soften the hardened wax buildup. After the wax is softened, you can use the syringe from the kit to gently cleanse your ear with clean, warm water. The wax should flow right out of your ears into the sink or shower. If you still notice a ringing noise, try some more drops and repeat the cleansing process.

If your ears become red and irritated, put the kit away and try it again the following day. Your ears aren't used to so much attention and might need a rest from the cleaning.

Removing normal amounts of wax from your ears can cause problems.

Taking away the fluid and its normal function can sometimes lead to dry ears. Your ears can become itchy due to the dryness. It can also lead to conditions such as swimmer's ear, because earwax helps to waterproof your ears. When you remove the oily coating, it can leave your ears unprotected.

Your doctor can clean the wax out of your ears if you have difficulty doing it yourself. Your doctor will also clean out your children's ears — special care should be taken with children because their ear canals are shorter than adults, and it is easy to damage the tender eardrum.

Never use your finger, a hairpin, a pencil, tweezers, sharp objects or even cotton swabs to clean your ears. Putting these things in your ear could push the wax deeper into your ear and even damage your eardrum.

Eye problems

4 ways to keep your eyes healthy

Being able to see the world around you is a precious gift. Here are four strategies to protect your eyes from illness or injury that could rob you of your sight.

Find relief for dry eyes. If you complain to your doctor of dry eyes or dry mouth, he might look for signs of congestive heart failure or even Parkinson's disease. These conditions are closely linked with these drying symptoms. Before you panic, talk to him about any over-the-counter or prescription medications you are taking. These could be the real source of your trouble. There are hundreds of drugs that can cause dry eyes and mouth, especially in older women. Painkillers and antidepressants are the two most common. Your doctor will probably suggest lubricating your eyes with saline drops. If this doesn't help, talk with him about changing your prescription.

See your doctor for the right diagnosis. You wake up with sore, red, crusty eyes. Is it an infection or allergies? Although it's best to see your doctor to be sure, here's what could be causing your problem.

- Bacterial conjunctivitis — Also known as pinkeye, this highly contagious infection can spread from one eye to the other and also to other people. Your doctor may prescribe drops or an ointment to reduce the infection time.

- Viral conjunctivitis — This usually shows up with a cold and, like a cold, won't get better with antibiotics. It generally runs its course in about a week. Since the virus spreads easily through touch, wash your hands, towels, pillowcases, and sheets often.

- Allergic conjunctivitis — This can be a reaction to pollen, pollution, mold, animals, smoke, or other allergens. It usually attacks both eyes and sometimes your nose and throat, too. You can take antihistamines or decongestants to relieve your symptoms.

Wet compresses, either warm or cold, may make you feel better, but don't use medicated drops designed to get rid of the red. While these will shrink the swollen blood vessels, making your eyes look white again, they haven't fixed what's really wrong. Remember, you don't want to just cover up this redness, which is often a sign of a more serious problem.

Handle contacts with care. Don't use bottled water to rinse, clean, or store your contact lenses. Experts tested 23 different brands of bottled water for various contaminants. Almost half of them contained live micro-organisms, like bacteria, yeasts, molds, amebae, and algae. Contacts washed in these bottled waters became contaminated within minutes. To avoid a serious eye infection, only use sterile contact lens solutions.

Practice proper makeup safety. Don't share makeup — especially eye products. Chemists analyzed over 3,000 cosmetics used by more than one person and found 10 percent contaminated with fungi. More than a hundred contained microorganisms that could cause disease. If a cosmetic contains preservatives, it's less likely to become contaminated, but there's still no guarantee. By passing around mascara or lipstick, you could be passing around germs and viruses.

• •
Faster relief from eye drops

Dropping medication into your eyes can be a frustrating and messy experience. You never know how much actually gets in your eye and stays there long enough to do any good. Follow these simple tips to make sure the medicine goes where it should.

- Lie, stand, or sit with your head tilted back. Look at the ceiling.

- Form a pocket for the medicine by gently pulling your lower lid out and down with two fingers.

- Don't look at the bottle. Squeeze a drop of medicine into the pocket. Never let the tip of the dropper touch you or any surface.

- Gently press on the inside corner of your closed eye for several minutes. This keeps the medicine from entering your tear duct.

- Blot away any excess with a tissue and repeat with the other eye, if necessary.

- Tell your doctor of any itching, burning, or puffiness.

• •

A multivitamin a day keeps cataracts away

Pop a multivitamin every morning and cut your risk of cataracts by a third. Sounds like a great reason to balance out a healthy diet with a daily supplement.

If you think protecting your vision is important enough to make a multivitamin part of your daily routine, be sure it contains these particular nutrients. In clinical research, they proved to be especially protective against cataracts.

Vitamin E. Experts are still examining the relationship between vitamin E and cataracts, but they say a supplement is a smart idea. Here's the evidence.

- People with low levels of vitamin E have a high rate of cataracts. And the opposite is true, as well — high levels of vitamin E accompany fewer cataracts.

- Those who take vitamin E supplements cut their risk in half.

- Nuclear cataracts, the most common kind, grow twice as fast in people who don't take vitamin E supplements when compared with people who do.

Some researchers say you can safely take up to 400 international units (IU) of vitamin E daily. To get more vitamin E in your diet, add a little wheat germ oil, sunflower seeds, or dried almonds. And instead of white flour and white rice, eat whole wheat, oats, and brown rice.

Vitamin C. The lens of your eye contains a high concentration of ascorbic acid, also known as vitamin C. Keeping your lens healthy is a good step toward better vision.

- In a test group of 4,000 seniors, those who got more vitamin C were less likely to have cataracts.

- Researchers studied nurses between the ages of 56 and 71. They found that those who took a vitamin C supplement for 10 years or more were 77 percent less likely to have even mild clouding of the lenses, compared with those who didn't take supplements. The advantage wasn't as great for those who supplemented for less than 10 years, however. It seems the amount of vitamin C in the supplement is less important than the number of years you take it.

To get more vitamin C from food, eat kiwis, oranges, lemons, tangerines, grapefruit, strawberries, broccoli, brussels sprouts, and sweet red peppers.

A multivitamin is especially important to eye health if you restrict your diet in any way. People on strict vegetarian diets — no animal products at all — are especially vulnerable to permanent vision loss unless they supplement with B1, B12, A, C, D, E, zinc, and selenium.

More natural ways to discourage cataracts

Cataracts are the leading cause of blindness. Half of all Americans have cataracts by age 50, and by age 75, that number increases to 70 percent. While age is the number one cause of cataracts, there are lifestyle choices you can make to decrease your risk.

Protect your eyes from the sun. Experts agree — if you spend too much time in the sun without protecting your eyes, you're at higher risk of developing eye diseases, like cataracts.

When buying sunglasses, select a pair that block at least 99 percent of ultraviolet (UV) light. If the label says "UV absorption up to 400 nm," that means the same thing. Don't worry about protection from infrared light. Research hasn't shown any connection between eye problems and the relatively low levels found in sunlight.

Amber, polarized, and mirrored lenses can make a difference in how well you see during different outdoor activities, but they don't have anything to do with protecting you from UV radiation. Neither does the color of the lenses nor how dark they are. Large, wrap-around styles are a good idea. They protect from all angles. Ordinary frames allow light to shine around the sides, over the tops, and into your eyes.

And remember — expensive doesn't necessarily mean better. You don't have to pay big bucks for good sunglasses. That $100 pair may have more style, but the $10 pair could be just as good, or better, for your eyes. UV protection is what matters most, not the price.

To judge the quality of sunglasses, it helps to look at something with a rectangular pattern — like floor tile. Hold the glasses several inches from your face, cover one eye, and move the glasses from side to side and up and down. The lines should stay straight. Choose another pair if the lines look wavy, especially in the center.

If you take medication that makes your skin more sensitive to the sun, your eyes will be more sensitive, too. These photosensitizing drugs include tetracycline, doxycycline, and allopurinol. Talk to your ophthalmologist if you have any questions.

Stay away from cigarettes. Cigarette smoke can do more than cloud up a room. It can dim your eyesight as well. While experts may not be able to explain how it happens, they do know smokers are two to three times more likely to get cataracts than non-smokers. Still, it's never too late to turn things around. By simply cutting out cigarettes, you'll be cutting your risk of cataracts, too.

Be aware of the aspirin controversy. Aspirin therapy for cataracts is still a controversial subject. While some studies indicate that taking aspirin might help prevent cataracts, more recent research shows long-term use of aspirin can actually increase your risk. Experts found that people who took one or more aspirin tablets a week for a period of 10 years were twice as likely to have cataracts as those who didn't take aspirin very often. This seemed to be truest for people under age 65.

In another large study, researchers found no evidence that taking low doses of aspirin every other day helped prevent cataracts. There is a possibility, however, that a treatment like this could decrease the number of required cataract surgeries — a $2.5 billion annual expense in the U.S. If aspirin therapy was able to postpone the need for surgery by several years, it could save millions of dollars in hospital bills.

A word of caution — if you are taking aspirin for your heart or other health reasons, don't stop without your doctor's approval.

Ask your doctor about estrogen. Post-menopausal women are at especially high risk of developing cataracts. Animal studies at the Indiana University School of Medicine show hormone replacement therapy might help prevent cataracts in older women.

Say no to alcohol. Scientists have found where there is regular alcohol use, there is also a slightly higher rate of cataracts. And having a daily drink is a greater risk than drinking just once a month. While researchers continue to study this connection, you might want to cut back on the alcohol.

Save your sight with leafy greens

Not since Popeye's bulging muscles has there been a better reason to add spinach to your menu. This green, leafy vegetable, along with kale, broccoli and collard greens, contains carotenoids — the newest superheroes in the fight against vision loss.

Carotenoids give brightly colored fruits and vegetables their vivid colors. Many of them act as antioxidants, fighting cell damage caused by UV light and free radicals. Two of these antioxidants, lutein and zeaxanthin, are particularly abundant in your eyes, protecting the delicate eye tissues from harm.

People who have cataracts and age-related macular degeneration (AMD) often have low levels of these two important antioxidants. This prompted researchers to find out if there's a connection.

In a 12-year study of over 70,000 women, those who ate the most lutein and zeaxanthin-containing foods, like spinach and kale, were 22 percent less likely to develop cataracts severe enough to require surgery.

Researchers in a multi-center Eye Disease Case-Control Study found that the people who ate the most carotenoids had a 43 percent lower risk of developing AMD. Spinach and collard greens, which are rich in lutein and zeaxanthin, were specifically associated with this lower risk.

In other research, of all the foods tested, broccoli and spinach lowered the risk of cataracts the most.

For all-round good health, eat lots of fruits and vegetables rich in carotenoids every day. But to give your eyes a little extra defense, go for the green.

100 grams (about 1/4 lb.)	micrograms of lutein and zeaxanthin
Kale (raw)	39,550
Kale (cooked)	15,798
Spinach (raw)	11,938
Turnip greens (fresh, cooked)	8,440
Collards (fresh, cooked)	8,091
Spinach (fresh, cooked)	7,043
Lettuce (romaine)	2,635
Broccoli (fresh)	2,226
Zucchini (raw)	2,125
Corn (fresh)	1,800
Cornmeal	1,355
Peas (canned)	1,350

100 grams (about 1/4 lb.)	micrograms of lutein and zeaxanthin
Brussels sprouts	1,290
Corn (canned)	884
Persimmons (Japanese)	834
Green beans (fresh)	700
Okra (cooked)	390
Carrots (raw, baby)	358
Lettuce (iceberg)	352
Cabbage (raw)	310
Celery (raw)	232
Orange	187
Peaches (raw)	57
Peaches (canned)	33

Rx for computer-weary eyes

Computers can bring information to you in seconds and put you in touch with people all over the world. But they can also make your neck ache, your head pound, your shoulders tense, and your eyes sore.

Eyestrain can be caused by poor posture, bad lighting, and an awkward workspace. It can also mean you need special computer glasses. If your glasses aren't designed for computer work, you may hold your head and body in positions that cause muscle and eye stress.

Practice these tips to keep your eyes safely fixed on the future.

See an eye doctor. Don't rely on drugstore computer glasses. Get a proper eye exam and an individual prescription.

Take a break. Get up and do something else for about 15 minutes for every 45 you spend at the computer.

Think about blinking. When you stare at a screen, you don't blink as often, and your eyes become dry. Studies show that dry eyes can lead to weak eyes, eye pain, headache, and dimmed vision.

Dribble some drops. Use a lubricating eye drop or tear replacement for dry or itchy eyes.

Get rid of the glare. Make sure there is no light reflecting on your computer screen. Move lamps, put up window blinds, or buy a glare reduction filter for your screen.

Do away with dust. Clean your screen often with a lint-free cloth.

Pick the proper palette. Choose a light screen with dark letters. This is easiest on the eyes.

Measure the distance. Position your computer screen carefully. It should be 4 to 9 inches below eye-level and 20 to 26 inches from your eyes.

Whether you are e-mailing your grandkids, shopping, or tracing your family history, see your doctor if you develop:

- tired, sore, or dry eyes
- blurred vision
- headaches
- difficulty focusing
- red, burning, or watery eyes
- changes in how you see colors

Fibromyalgia

Here's how to cope with symptoms

You're in pain almost all the time. You can't sleep. You feel bone-aching fatigue. You've been to numerous doctors, had a battery of tests, and you still don't know what's wrong with you.

For the estimated three to six million people with fibromyalgia, that's pretty typical. It can take as long as two years for your doctor to reach a diagnosis because so many other conditions have to be ruled out first.

To help guide doctors in identifying this confusing syndrome, the American College of Rheumatology set criteria for the diagnosis of fibromyalgia. These criteria include the presence of widespread pain for at least three months; pain in specific areas of your spine, chest, or lower back; and pain in at least 11 of 18 tender spots upon pressure.

Besides these symptoms, most people with fibromyalgia experience fatigue, insomnia, and morning stiffness. Other problems include irritable bowel syndrome, headache, Raynaud syndrome-type symptoms, and psychological problems.

If you think you may have fibromyalgia, talk with your doctor. Nonsteroidal anti-inflammatory drugs (NSAIDs) and other pain relievers, antidepressants, and muscle relaxants can be used to treat this painful condition.

Exercise. This may be one of the most effective treatments for fibromyalgia, even though it may cause pain and discomfort at first. Choose the low-impact aerobic type, such as swimming, riding a stationary bike, or using a ski-type machine. Start slowly and build up to at least 20 to 30 minutes of exercise four or more times a week. Then, if you like, you can move to high-impact exercises, such as walking, running, or tennis.

Manage stress. Stress can be a trigger for fibromyalgia. Decide on your priorities and eliminate the things that are not really important to you. Stress-management techniques, like biofeedback, meditation, and relaxation, can help you learn to deal with your stress and your pain.

Don't lose sleep. Getting too little sleep can aggravate your symptoms. You probably know you shouldn't drink coffee, tea, or colas before going to bed. They contain caffeine, which is a stimulant, and can keep you awake. You may not realize that nicotine in cigarettes is also a stimulant. And although drinking alcohol can make you sleepy, it can also cause you to wake up during the night.

Don't overdo it. Try to plan your activities. Don't do too much one day and end up having a bad day the next.

Find support. It always helps to know you're not alone. Joining a fibromyalgia support group will give you an opportunity to talk with other people and share ideas. Your local chapter of The Arthritis Foundation can help you find a support group.

Encouraging news for sufferers

People with fibromyalgia face a daily battle against the pain and fatigue caused by this poorly understood syndrome. To make matters worse, they often have to battle the misperceptions of other people who think their illness is "all in their heads."

Mental problems, like depression and stress, often go along with fibromyalgia, but most experts agree those are symptoms of the physical syndrome, rather than the other way around.

The latest research is encouraging. Scientists at the University of Florida have found that people with fibromyalgia have an abnormal central nervous system response to ordinary repetitive touches.

Researchers tested people with and without fibromyalgia by repeatedly placing warm plates on their arms. The people without fibromyalgia felt the plates but reported no pain from the sensation. The people with fibromyalgia, however, began to feel more and more pain each time the plates were placed on them, until the pain was unbearable.

While this study still doesn't explain why people get fibromyalgia, it does lend credibility to fibromyalgia as a physical syndrome, and it leads to greater understanding. Researchers are continuing to study fibromyalgia at the University of Florida and elsewhere.

Food poisoning

Foolproof formula for foiling food poisoning

Prevent the nausea, stomach pain, and diarrhea of food poisoning by remembering these four steps — clean, quarantine, cook, and chill.

Clean:

- If you plan to eat fruits and vegetables raw, wash them carefully.

- After handling raw meat, wash your hands, utensils, and your cutting board in hot, soapy water.

- Use paper towels.

- Sanitize your sponge by running it through the dishwasher and then zapping it in the microwave for several minutes.

- Disinfect your kitchen sink, drain, and disposal by pouring in a mixture of one teaspoon of chlorine bleach and one quart of water. Do this at least once a week.

- Use bleach or commercial cleaners containing bleach to sanitize your kitchen counters.

- Wash the tops of cans with soap and water before you open them.

- Wash the can opener blade every time you use it.

- Rubber gloves can harbor bacteria, too. Wash them often with hot water and soap or bleach.

Quarantine:

- Don't let raw meat or raw juices come in contact with other foods.

- Use separate cutting boards for meats and vegetables.

- Don't put cooked meat, poultry, or seafood back onto the same plate that held it raw.

- When marinating meat, don't use any leftover marinade as a baste or sauce without boiling it first.

Cook:

- Heat ready-to-eat meats, like hot dogs, thoroughly.

- If you aren't eating take-out food immediately, say within a couple of hours, reheat it to steaming hot temperatures. Don't simply keep it warm since this is the perfect environment for bacteria to grow. Microwaving carry-out food is the best way to kill bacteria.

- Reheat leftovers to 165 degrees Fahrenheit or until bubbling hot.

- When in doubt, use a meat thermometer. This is especially important when grilling. Meats tend to brown quickly on the outside but can still be uncooked on the inside.

- Stir and rotate microwaved foods to make sure they are heated evenly. Let them stand the required amount of time to finish cooking.

- Never eat hamburgers that are still pink inside. Order them well-done.

Chill:

- Don't leave perishable foods at room temperature for longer than two hours.

- Your refrigerator should be set at 40 degrees Fahrenheit (or less) and your freezer at 0 degrees. Use an appliance thermometer to be sure. You may have to lower these settings in the summer.

- Thaw and marinate foods in the refrigerator, never on the counter or at room temperature.

• •
Shop smart to keep food safe

To protect your family and your dinner guests, follow these basic rules of food safety.

- Shop for packaged and canned foods first.

- Don't buy bulging or dented cans or cracked jars. Make sure all lids are tightly sealed.

- Check expiration dates and the "use by" or "sell by" date on dairy products. Pick the one that will stay fresh longest in your refrigerator.

- Only buy refrigerated eggs. Open each carton and make sure the eggs are clean and unbroken.

- Pick up your frozen foods and perishables, such as meat, poultry, and fish last. Always put these products in separate plastic bags so drippings don't contaminate other food in your shopping cart.

- Don't buy frozen food if the package is open, torn, or crushed. Make sure the product is solidly frozen.

- Check for cleanliness at the meat and fish counters and the salad bar. For instance, cooked shrimp lying on the same bed of ice as raw fish could become contaminated.

- Don't buy shellfish from vendors at roadside stands or selling from the back of a truck.

• If it will take you more than an hour to get your groceries home, take an ice chest in your car to keep frozen and perishable foods cold.

● ●

Sure-fire ways to dodge *Salmonella*

Approximately one egg in 20,000 contains *Salmonella* bacteria. If that egg is not thoroughly cooked, it will make someone very sick, perhaps even kill them. There are two ways to prevent this from happening — educate people on the safe handling and cooking of eggs and eliminate *Salmonella* from all eggs.

Get the hard-boiled facts. On average, you will eat over 200 eggs this year. Will every one of them be fully cooked? Have you ever let your grandkids eat raw cookie dough? Do you love your eggs sunny side up? If you don't cook an egg long enough to set the yolk, *Salmonella* bacteria may still be alive.

The Food and Drug Administration (FDA) is trying to help. They are requiring a new safe handling label on all eggs that have not been treated to destroy bacteria. It says:

"Eggs may contain harmful bacteria known to cause serious illness, especially in children, the elderly, and persons with weakened immune systems. For your protection: keep eggs refrigerated, cook eggs until yolks are firm, and cook foods containing eggs thoroughly."

Break the bacteria cycle. *Salmonella* is passed from an infected chicken to her eggs. Once a hen tests positive for *Salmonella*, her eggs should only be used in products like ice cream, pasta, mayonnaise, and baked goods — items that are pasteurized. This means they have been heated until all bacteria are killed.

The FDA is proposing a federal law requiring that all eggs and egg products be kept at 45 degrees Fahrenheit or less, a temperature that prevents the growth of bacteria. This would include stores, restaurants, delis, caterers, vending machines, hospitals, nursing homes, schools, and even the vehicles used to transport eggs. Check your refrigerator's temperature and be careful how you store eggs.

Look to the future. Be on the lookout for a brand of eggs that have been pasteurized while still in the shell. This revolutionary idea, patented by Davidson's Pasteurized Eggs, allows you to eat these special eggs lightly cooked, or even raw, without the fear of developing food poisoning. Approved by the U.S. Department of Agriculture, these eggs should be available soon. They will cost a bit more, but that's a small price to pay for peace of mind.

● ●
Pet treats harbor hidden danger

Fido loves those smoky chew treats — pig and cow ears, beef chews, hooves, dried strips, and braided chews — but they may contain a hidden danger, the bacteria *Salmonella*. They won't hurt Fido, but you could get sick, very sick. In fact, you could become infected just by handling the treats.

Symptoms are similar to the flu and include nausea, vomiting, diarrhea, and stomach pain. Children, seniors, and people with weak immune systems are especially vulnerable and should avoid handling the pet treats. For everyone else, prevention is fairly simple. Just wash your hands with soap and water after touching the treats. At least 30 cases of *Salmonella* poisoning in Canada were traced back to pig ear dog chews, prompting the FDA to restrict the import of these pet treats until the problem is resolved.

● ●

Don't let mold spoil your meal

Have you ever found a bit of green, fuzzy stuff on your favorite cheese or on a piece of bread? Perhaps you pinched off the bad part and ate the rest. Moldy foods are usually considered an irritation, not a health hazard, like *E. coli*, *Salmonella*, and other bacteria. The truth is — some molds produce mycotoxins, poisons that can be very dangerous. These hardy toxins can survive a long time in food, can grow in refrigerator temperatures, and aren't destroyed by cooking.

Mold is a plant, consisting of roots, a stalk, and seeds called spores. The stalk and the spores give mold its distinctive look and color and also spread the mold from one place to another. You can't see the roots, but they can extend far down inside a food and are, surprisingly, the most dangerous part of mold. This is where the toxins are produced. If you simply remove only the visible portion of the mold, you are leaving behind the real health hazard.

Know when to toss and when to trim. If you find mold on these foods, throw them away:

bacon	bananas
berries	bread
cake	canned ham
cottage cheese	cucumbers
fresh corn	hot dogs
jelly	leftovers
lettuce	lunch meat
melons	pastries
peaches	peanut butter
rolls	soft cheese (mozzarella, brie)
sour cream	spinach
tomatoes	yogurt

If you find mold on the following foods, simply trim at least an inch deep and eat or re-cover with clean wrap. If your knife touches the mold, you will spread the spores through the rest of the food.

apples	bell peppers
broccoli	brussels sprouts
cabbage	carrots
cauliflower	garlic
hard cheese (Cheddar, Swiss)	onions
pears	potatoes
turnips	zucchini

Fight fungus fast and efficiently. Control mold spores inside your refrigerator by cleaning it out regularly. Wash the inside with a solution of baking soda and water, rinse, then dry. Wipe off any mold on the door's rubber seals with bleach and water. Don't allow food — especially produce — to sit in your refrigerator too long. And last, but not least, don't sniff moldy foods. You can inhale the spores and develop respiratory problems.

If you are really unsure about a certain food's safety, call the U.S. Department of Agriculture's Food Safety and Inspection Service Meat and Poultry Hotline. They can answer questions about all kinds of perishable foods.

1-800-535-4555 (Toll-free nationwide)

(202) 720-3333 (Washington, D.C. area)

1-800-256-7072 (TDD/TTY)

• •
Cinnamon clobbers deadly *E. coli*

Fall is a time of cool weather, pumpkins, and apple cider, but buying a gallon of fresh apple juice from a roadside stand is not a safe way to end an October day.

Unpasteurized apple juice is very likely to contain *E. coli*, one of the deadliest strains of bacteria known to man. Yet, a simple spice may be the strongest weapon against this dangerous bug.

In tests performed at Kansas State University, cinnamon knocked out heavy doses of *E. coli* added to apple juice. The more cinnamon, the less *E. coli*. When it was added along with commercial preservatives, the *E. coli* bacteria virtually disappeared within three days.

Despite this good news, don't swirl a cinnamon stick in your juice and think you're safe from *E. coli*. Experts aren't recommending an exact method just yet. For the time being, select pasteurized apple juice and add cinnamon just for good taste.

• •

Safest way to eat sprouts

Seed sprouts may seem like the perfect health food — fresh, raw, natural, and jam-packed with nutrients. Every year, about 300,000 tons of these veggies are eaten by health-conscious people throughout the United States. Unfortunately, along with hefty doses of vitamins and minerals, they may be getting a shot of disease-causing bacteria, like *E. coli* and *Salmonella*.

The problem of contaminated sprouts is so widespread that scientists at the Food and Drug Administration (FDA) and the Centers for Disease Control and Prevention (CDC) are telling some people to stop eating sprouts completely. According to these experts, the young, the old, and those with weak immune systems are at risk of developing serious illnesses from sprout contamination.

Reports of food-borne illnesses from soy, cress, alfalfa, wheat, radish, mustard, clover, and mung bean sprouts have occurred worldwide since the early 1970s. But only recently have experts collected and studied the information.

Authorities have traced the outbreaks to several strains of bacteria from many processing plants in different parts of the world. Contamination usually begins with the seeds, which can become infected almost anywhere along the way. Once the seeds are contaminated, you can't do anything to keep the sprouts safe. And it's not only a concern for commercially grown sprouts. Homegrown sprouts from contaminated seeds will be contaminated, even if they're grown under clean conditions.

To combat the problem, the FDA has tested alcohol, heat, water, radiation, and chemicals. As yet, they have found no guaranteed way to kill the bacteria without irreversibly damaging the seeds. However, they are considering two possibilities:

1) a required warning label on sprout packages and instructions for safe handling

2) a voluntary quality assurance program where sprout growers who follow sanitation guidelines and have their facilities inspected could label their products as ISGA (International Sprout Growers Association) certified

In the meantime, if you are a healthy adult and choose to eat sprouts, follow these tips:

- Buy only refrigerated sprouts. Choose ones that look crisp and have the buds attached. Avoid sprouts that are slimy, dark, or smell musty. Although you can't tell by looking at them if they've been contaminated, at least you'll be choosing fresh sprouts.

- At home, keep your sprouts refrigerated (at less than 40

degrees Fahrenheit). Bacteria thrive in warm, damp environments.

- Rinse sprouts thoroughly with water before eating them. This will not remove bacteria, but it will help remove surface dirt. Unfortunately, sprouts grown from contaminated seeds will have bacteria inside.

- Cook your sprouts to reduce the risk.

If you develop diarrhea, stomach cramps, and fever after eating sprouts, tell your doctor immediately. Some bacteria, like *Salmonella* and *E. coli*, can be extremely dangerous.

13 ways to build a better bug trap

Modern technology is wonderful, but in some cases, high-tech just makes matters worse. Take bugs. Most people find them annoying, if not downright unacceptable. They hate the way bugs fly, crawl, sting, bite, and spread germs. Enter technology and the bug zapper is born.

This device attracts pesky flying insects and electrocutes them into oblivion — at least that's the idea. The truth is, only a very small percentage of the "zapped" insects are true pests, while all kinds of good bugs are exterminated. Besides that, research shows a zapper will draw insects to the area then won't always kill them. You are much more likely to be bitten by a mosquito near a zapper than anywhere else. And what really happens to the zapped bug is enough to send you running from the picnic table. Any virus or bacteria that is on, or in, the insect is sprayed up to 6 feet away. (The average housefly carries about 2 million bacteria, including cholera and typhoid.) In addition, microscopic insect parts are sent swirling through the air where you and your family could breathe them in.

If this is making you feel a bit queasy, here are some safer, more natural alternatives for controlling pests in your home and yard.

- Buy body products with citronella, like lotions and soaps, or citronella candles to burn outside. Citronella oil comes from a perennial grass of the same name. It has a light, lemony fragrance and is proven to repel insects.

- Combine one pint of milk, a quarter pound of raw sugar, and 2 ounces of ground pepper in a saucepan. Simmer the mixture for about 10 minutes. Pour into shallow dishes, and set around your house or patio. Flies will flock to this treat and drown.

- Wipe down your countertops, cabinets, and floors with a solution of one part vinegar to one part water to keep ants away.

- Squeeze lemon juice in the holes or cracks where ants are getting into your house. Slice the lemon peel and scatter it around the entrance to make sure they get the hint.

- Find out where ants are entering and create your own homemade barrier. Ants usually will not cross a line of bone meal, powdered charcoal, cream of tartar, red chili pepper, paprika, or dried peppermint.

- Make your own ant traps. Use one cup of clear corn syrup and a half cup of warm water. Microwave for 40 seconds and stir to blend. Add two teaspoons of boric acid powder to the mixture and stir. Find some shallow containers (like bottle caps or small pieces of aluminum foil, bent up at the edges) and pour some of this mixture in them. Set these "traps" where you see ants but out of the reach of children and pets.

- Scratch the peel of an orange and leave it out. Citrus repels flies. You can also hang a bundle of cloves, or keep a pot of fresh mint in your kitchen window to keep flies away.

- Sprinkle borax or dry soap in the bottom of your garbage can after it's washed and dried to keep flies away.

- Make your own fly paper by boiling sugar, corn syrup, and water. Spread the sticky mixture on brown paper, and lay it out or hang it where it will attract flies.

- To repel fleas, grow a pot of basil in your kitchen window. Water it regularly from the bottom for a stronger smell. It works just as well to put crushed, dried basil leaves in small bowls or hang some in muslin bags.

- Control roaches by scattering a mixture of equal parts baking soda and powdered sugar in the infested area. The sugar attracts them, and the baking soda kills them. Or repel these creepy critters by cutting hedge apples (Osage oranges) in half and placing them in your cabinets, in your basement, or under your house.

- Combine half a cup of borax with one-fourth cup of flour. Put it in a jar. Punch holes in the lid and sprinkle it along baseboards and door sills. Or try a combination of oatmeal, flour, and plaster of Paris. Put it in dishes in areas where roaches are likely to hide. Take care that no pets or children will get into either of these mixtures. Borax is toxic if eaten.

- Put saucers of inexpensive red wine under the cabinets. Roaches crawl in, drink it, get tipsy, and drown.

Foot problems

7 ways to stomp out athlete's foot

Athlete's foot isn't just for athletes. It's for anyone who provides this fungus with a perfect environment to grow — warm, moist feet. If you wear tight shoes and socks, especially in a warm climate, or don't dry your feet promptly and completely after bathing, you're the perfect target for an athlete's foot attack.

Symptoms can vary from simple redness and a rash on the bottom and sides of your feet to blisters and cracked and peeling skin between your toes. Some people develop toenail infections that cause the nail to split or even fall off.

To prevent this uncomfortable condition, try these tips:

- Wash your feet every day and dry them completely. Pay special attention to the skin between your toes.

- Don't wear tight shoes and heavy socks. Sandals are great but going barefoot is even better.

- Choose socks made from a natural fiber, like cotton, which will draw moisture away from your skin. If your socks get sweaty, change them as soon as you can.

- Sprinkle anti-fungal powder into your shoes now and then. It helps keep them dry and will attack any fungus that may be hiding out.

- If you spend time in locker rooms or other such places, don't walk around with bare feet. Get yourself some shower shoes or flip-flops.

- Toss out any shoes you wore without socks while you had the fungus. This will help prevent reinfection.

- Every once in a while, rub some anti-fungal cream between your toes, over your nails, and on the bottoms of your feet. It will form a barrier against bacteria, yeasts, and fungi while soothing and protecting your skin. Or try a zinc oxide-based diaper rash ointment to provide a waterproof coating on your feet.

There are plenty of over-the-counter anti-fungal creams to help treat this itchy pest. But before you go self-medicating, make sure the rash on your foot is really athlete's foot. It could be something else and using the wrong medication could make the problem worse.

If you have a really stubborn or severe case, ask your doctor for help. He can prescribe foot soaks or oral medication. But remember to keep using your medication even after the symptoms disappear. This will make sure you get rid of all the fungus.

• •
The power of a foot massage

The next time you're feeling a little ragged around the edges or uncomfortable from a headache or muscle strain, try a foot massage. Who would have thought having your feet pampered could make you forget about the aches and pains in other parts of your body — but clinical studies say it's true.

In a group of women undergoing outpatient surgery, half received a foot massage and painkillers after the procedure and half received just the medication. Those with the tickled tootsies said they felt less pain.

So put up your feet and let someone rub your pain away.
• •

New procedure relieves heel pain

If you suffer from heel pain or heel spurs, you may have tried cortisone injections, worn special shoe inserts, or performed unusual exercises. You may even have had surgery. Sometimes these treatments work — sometimes they don't. If you're still living with heel pain, talk with your doctor about a new treatment called shock wave therapy.

The idea comes from a tried and true remedy for kidney and gallbladder stones. Using highly concentrated sound waves from outside your body, a device called a lithotriptor disintegrates these stones — without risk, surgery, or side effects.

Now doctors are experimenting with this same procedure on other conditions, like heel spurs and tendinitis. The concept is the same, but the goal and use of the device are somewhat different. With orthotripsy, doctors use a similar machine but release a much lower dose of energy. The shock waves simply alert your body that an injured area needs attention. The healing process kicks in, and your body begins repairing damaged tissues and growing new bone.

The FDA has not yet approved the device for this kind of shock wave therapy, but clinical trials have had good results. The success rate for heel spurs has been an amazing 90 percent.

This revolutionary treatment can be used for tendinitis, plantar fasciitis, pseudarthrosis, and golf or tennis elbow, and it may, in the future, combat osteoporosis by increasing bone density.

Gallstones

Stop problems before they start

Gallstones affect more and more people every year. And here's why — more and more people are overweight, getting less exercise, and eating not-so-healthy food.

If you want to lower your risk of developing gallstones, here are some things you can do:

Work out an exercise program. If you need another reason to lace up your tennis shoes, here it is — physical activity will reduce your risk of developing gallstones. You don't have to train for the next marathon, just start some kind of recreation that gets your blood flowing. Walk, bike, swim, or take that dance class at the "Y." Just two or three hours a week can cut your risk by 20 percent. On the other hand, research shows the more hours you spend sitting in front of the TV, the greater your risk of gallstones.

Fill up your cup. No one ever says anything good about coffee — except that it may help you stay awake through that boring meeting. But now, researchers at the Harvard School of Public Health say there's something about coffee that positively mugs gallstones. Men who drink two or three cups a day have fewer gallstones than noncoffee drinkers. And men who drink more than four are even better off.

It doesn't matter whether it's percolated, drip, or instant. It just has to be caffeinated. Decaf coffee and sodas and teas containing caffeine don't provide the same benefit.

Experts think coffee not only gets your gallbladder and intestines moving, it also lowers the amount of cholesterol in your bile, which turns into gallstones. Don't start drinking coffee just to ward off gallstones, but if you're already hooked on "joe," you may be doing your gallbladder some good.

Add soy to your menu. Replacing animal protein in your diet with soy protein could be the newest strategy in the war on gallstones. If you think about this, it makes sense. Gallstones are made from cholesterol. Cholesterol comes mainly from animal fat. Foods high in animal fat, like bacon, hot dogs, sausage, egg yolks, shellfish, and dairy products, are also high in cholesterol. When you cut out the source of cholesterol, you eliminate the gallstones. This may explain why vegetarians, on average, have fewer stones. You won't get rid of existing gallstones this way, but you may be stopping future problems.

So how do you get more soy in your diet? Don't be intimidated by your supermarket's health food section. Walk around and explore. Try new foods. You'll find lots of meatless products made with soy, including soy burgers, hot dogs, margarine, cream cheese, and soy milk.

Soy flour is another great way to boost the protein content of your home-cooked breads, muffins, and cakes. Try replacing up to 25 percent of a recipe's white or wheat flour content with soy flour. (Don't use 100 percent soy flour in recipes that include yeast because the dough won't rise properly.) And try this egg substitute — one tablespoon of soy flour plus one tablespoon of water equals one whole egg, with no cholesterol.

While you're shopping, get to know tofu, probably the most well-know soybean product. It usually comes in block form and has about the same weight and consistency as a soft cheese. You can cut these blocks into strips or cubes for use in stir fries or soups, or you can blend them into shakes and salad dressings.

One of the remarkable properties of tofu is that it has almost no taste. Instead, it absorbs the flavor of whatever it is cooked with. You can use tofu as a substitute wherever meat, cheese, or yogurt is called for. Or simply add a few cubes to a recipe to give it an extra, healthful kick.

Tofu comes in several textures, ranging from soft to extra firm. Be sure to buy the right kind for the type of cooking you want to do. For example, extra firm tofu works best for grilling, while softer varieties are better suited for blending into dressings.

Nutritionists recommend that you buy refrigerated, individually wrapped tofu because it has less chance of being contaminated. At home, tofu will keep in your refrigerator for up to a week. Keep it submerged in water, and change the water once a day. Keep in mind that some brands of tofu can be high in fat, so be label conscious when you're shopping. Low-fat varieties are almost always available.

Look for tempeh, miso, and powdered soy protein, too. These are all good ways to get more soy and prevent gallstones.

Consider a new medicine. The first medication to prevent gallstones is now on the market. Its generic name is ursodiol, but it is currently marketed under the brand name Actigall. It helps dissolve gallstones and is a good alternative if surgery is not a safe choice for you. It's also especially helpful if you are obese and losing weight rapidly, a situation that puts you at high risk for developing gallstones.

Actigall does not fix a bad situation quickly. It could take months for this drug to completely dissolve your gallstones. Your doctor can tell you if Actigall is something you should consider.

(New research claims soy may accelerate brain aging. For more information, see the *Mental impairment* chapter.)

●●●●●●●●●●●●●●●●●●●●●●●●●●●

Outsmart gallstones with apple juice?

Are you willing to try an unusual home remedy for your gall-stones? A chemical engineer wrote into the prestigious medical journal, *The Lancet*, with a self-treatment that he claimed worked on his wife's gallstones.

She drank one liter of apple juice every day for a week. On the seventh night, she drank a cup of olive oil just before bedtime, then slept on her left side all night. The next morning, she passed her gallstones.

While there is no scientific evidence to support this treatment, it is a fairly safe, gentle option. Just be sure and talk with your doctor before trying it.

●●●●●●●●●●●●●●●●●●●●●●●●●

Dodge stones with peppermint

The old folk remedy of drinking peppermint tea to soothe your upset stomach is actually an accepted remedy for several intestinal problems. But did you know peppermint can help prevent painful gallstones?

Distinguished herbalists and the American Botanical Council agree that peppermint has certain properties that cause your gall-bladder to release more bile into the intestines. This serves to flush out your gallbladder, making it less likely that stones will form. It can even dislodge those you already have.

In one study, almost half of the people with gallstones successfully treated them with peppermint. These people had complete remission within two years.

Although a cup of hot peppermint tea will probably make you feel better, a more effective form is enteric-coated peppermint oil capsules. You can find these in your health food store. Be sure to talk with your doctor before you use peppermint to treat your gallstones.

Hair and nail troubles

Turn heads with these hair-care hints

Looking good doesn't have to take a lot of time or money. To keep your hair healthy and beautiful, try these winning tips.

Clean your combs. Your brushes and combs will keep your hair cleaner and healthier if you sanitize them regularly. Soak them every week in hot water plus one-fourth cup baking soda.

Don't throw money down the drain. Taking care of your hair the way the hair care industry says you should can be both expensive and time consuming. But is it really necessary? Many experts don't think so. Plain water and an inexpensive shampoo are all most people really need.

Any shampoo will take care of the natural oils your scalp produces, and rinsing with plain water washes away the dead skin cells that cause dandruff. If you feel like expensive, protein-packed shampoos make your hair more manageable, that's fine. Just remember, from a health standpoint, your hair will be perfectly healthy without them. And your wallet might feel better, too.

Stretch your shampoo. Don't throw out your shampoo when it's down to that last bit in the bottom. Just add water until the bottle is about one-third full. Shake it up a bit and squeeze onto your hair. You'll use almost every drop.

Choose a conditioner that's right for you. Your drugstore's display of hair conditioners can confound and confuse you, but don't get frustrated. Once you learn the difference between them, you'll know what bottle to buy.

- Cream rinses are a mixture of wax, thickeners, and chemicals called quaternary ammonium salts. This combination makes your hair easier to style and control. Cream rinses flatten the hair's cuticles and are excellent for hair that tangles easily. Just don't forget to rinse well.

- Instant conditioners are similar to cream rinses and usually are made of waxes, oils, emulsifiers, amino acids, keratin, collagen, balsam, and film-forming polymers. They coat each strand of hair to help repair damage. Instant conditioners don't rebuild the hair shaft, but they do fill in the cracks to help make each hair shaft whole. They also make your hair look fluffier and shinier.

- Deep conditioners are left on the hair for several minutes and then rinsed off. Sometimes heat is used on the hair after the conditioner is applied. Made from hydrolyzed proteins and film-forming agents, they are especially designed for dry and damaged hair. Apply a deep conditioner a few days before having your hair colored. This keeps your hair from drying out during the coloring process.

- Body builders are thin, clear fluids made up of water and plastic-like substances. They coat your hair and give it lift. However, some of these conditioners can end up drying out your hair or making oily hair even oilier.

- Hair repair products are actually absorbed by the hair shaft. These products bind with your hair and close up split ends.

Do away with dandruff. If the flakes are swirling around you like a blizzard — and it's only July — you need to get your dandruff under control. Some commercial products work and some don't. The next time you're choosing from among the rows of plastic bottles promising miracles, read the ingredients. If a product contains the anti-fungal tea tree oil, odds are you'll get great results.

If you want to try a home remedy, rinse your hair with lemon juice every day. You'll give dandruff flakes a citrus brushoff.

Fix the frizzies. If you've got wild hair, tame it with this easy recipe. Mix together one cup water and one cup vinegar. Pour this on your hair after you shampoo and condition. Allow the solution to set for two minutes before rinsing.

Go gentle with gray. Gray hair is more resistant to hair dyeing than any other color. That means your hair color may not "take" as well or last as long. But if you re-dye within a short period of time, you run the risk of damaging, breaking, and perhaps even losing your hair. Talk to a professional before you make a hair-raising mistake.

Highlight your assets. Are you thinking about going blonde, but the cost of a beauty salon treatment makes your hair stand on end? Consider making your own hair-streaking product. Get some alum, an aluminum compound, from your drugstore and mix it with just enough honey to form a thick paste. With your fingers, paint the mixture onto the strands of hair you want highlighted. Sit in the sun for about 45 minutes, then shampoo.

Let a student learn on your locks. You can get a good haircut, perm, or color treatment for bargain bucks at your local beauty or barber school. Check your yellow pages for these schools and call about their prices.

Relax your stresses and your tresses. A steam bath or a sauna can do more than make tired, achy muscles feel wonderful. It can give your hair a boost at the same time. Just apply conditioner and wrap your head in a warm, moist towel. Both your hair and your body will feel pampered.

Get rid of the green. Green hair from the chlorine in a swimming pool can be a real headache. Try some aspirin — but don't swallow them. Dissolve six to eight tablets in a glass of warm water. Pour it through your hair, saturating it completely. Leave it on for 10 minutes, then rinse thoroughly. Shampoo, rinse again, and the green should disappear.

Give hair loss the brush-off

Losing your hair is not just a cosmetic problem. It can affect your social and emotional well-being. Most people have trouble coping with hair loss. That's why billions of dollars are spent each year researching and marketing hair loss remedies. There are no miracle cures, just some things you might want to consider.

Amino acids. Arginine and cysteine are amino acids necessary for hair growth — your hair follicles need them to produce hair. Many people claim taking supplements strengthens their hair and nails. You can buy these as liquid supplements at health food stores.

Biotin and folic acid. Be careful with these two B vitamins. Granted, you do need them for your hair to grow, but most people get plenty from a normal diet. Unless you have too little because of another health condition, don't load up on supplements. Too much biotin and folic acid can actually cause your hair to fall out. A general multi-vitamin should fill in any nutritional gaps without causing problems for you.

Cosmetic aids. There are several cosmetic approaches that can make your hair look longer and thicker — at least temporarily. These hair additions are designed to be worn continuously for up to eight weeks. Both men and women can wear them while sleeping, bathing, and swimming. Hair additions can be applied several ways.

- Braiding — You can attach human or synthetic hair to your own hair with braids.

- Hair bonding — This technique requires gluing synthetic or human hair to your existing scalp hair.

- Hair integration — This popular approach involves hand-tying individual synthetic or human hair fibers to a crocheted web you wear on your scalp.

If you decide to try hair additions, be careful. While it is an easy way to hide hair loss, you could make matters worse. If your hair additions are too heavy or pull too tightly on your scalp, you can lose even more hair. Also, be sure to clean your natural hair and the hair additions properly to avoid scalp disease.

Gene therapy. Sometimes your own immune system attacks your hair follicles by mistake and causes your hair to stop growing or even fall out. Experts think they could correct the problem if they could find the genes responsible for this disorder. The goal of gene therapy is to replace the damaged genes or increase certain "good" genes that could stop this from happening.

At Cornell University, laboratory studies on animals show that gene therapy can cause hair growth. However, it hasn't yet been tested on humans.

Prescription drugs. Manufacturers of minoxidil, a drug applied to your scalp, claim it stops hair loss. Marketed under the brand name Rogaine, it was originally developed as a pill to treat high blood pressure, but it had an interesting side effect. It made hair grow thicker and longer. Although there are a number of possible explanations, experts believe it works by increasing blood flow.

Minoxidil seems to work best for young men with mild to moderate hair loss. The results for women using this treatment are not as remarkable. For minoxidil to work, you must use the product regularly for several years, and it may be weeks before you see any improvement. In addition, if you stop using minoxidil, not only will you stop growing new hair, any recently grown hair will fall out.

Minoxidil, which was originally quite expensive, is now available under several generic brands, making the price more reasonable.

Makers of the drug finasteride claim it can increase hair thickness and length and prevent hair loss. Its brand name is Propecia. Women should not use this drug. Studies show that pregnant women, or women planning to become pregnant, who are exposed to crushed or broken finasteride tablets risk exposing their male fetuses and causing birth defects.

There are similar drugs either on the market or in development by major pharmaceutical companies. Compresses, sprays, creams, and shampoos are available now and more are awaiting Food and Drug Administration (FDA) approval.

Zinc. Zinc is a mineral necessary for good health. The recommended dietary allowance (RDA) is 12 to 15 milligrams (mg). Studies have shown that people experiencing hair loss often have low levels of zinc. In addition, zinc lotions reduce the amount of oil on your scalp. In theory, this could unblock hair follicles, encouraging growth. However, there is no evidence that taking zinc or applying zinc to your scalp will encourage new hair growth. Keep in mind that too much zinc can actually make your hair fall out.

Other treatments. Devices that use electrical fields or energy wavelengths to stimulate hair growth don't seem to work as well as other treatments and are quite expensive. They also have not been approved by the FDA.

Be careful trying anything your doctor hasn't prescribed. Many unapproved treatments can cause serious side effects or interact dangerously with other medications.

The American Hair Loss Council is a nonprofit organization that publishes objective information for consumers. They focus on surgical and nonsurgical treatments for hair loss. Call 1-888-873-9719 for more information or visit their Web site <www.health-library.com/hairloss.html>.

Halt hair loss with herbs

Trying to choose from the slew of products claiming to restore hair is enough to make you want to pull your hair out, especially if you're looking for a natural treatment.

The Food and Drug Administration does not regulate herbal and over-the-counter remedies. Many products may seem similar, but they contain widely differing amounts of ingredients. Make sure you read labels and talk with your doctor or pharmacist for guidance. No one treatment is right for everyone. You may have to try several products before finding one that works for you. And finally, don't expect miracles. There is no overnight cure for hair loss.

Get expert help from essential oils. Treating hair loss with essential oils has been scientifically studied, and the results are clear — it works. In one study, 86 people suffering from alopecia areata, a specific kind of hair loss, massaged essential oils into their scalps every day.

The essential oils used — thyme, rosemary, lavender, and cedarwood — were mixed with jojoba and grapeseed oils. These "carrier" oils dilute the essential oils to prevent irritation. This combination improved hair growth for almost half of the people in just seven months.

Another mixture that claims to put hair back on your head includes lavender oil, calamus oil, gentian tincture, and rosemary spirits. Royal jelly and nettle may also stimulate hair growth.

Aromatherapy, or treating hair loss with essential oils, can be a safe and natural remedy, but do your homework. Check out your local library and bookstore for more information about essential oils, including exact recipes and important warnings.

See results with saw palmetto. While the herb saw palmetto (*serenoa repens*) has been proven to treat prostate problems in men, it has not been studied for treating hair loss. Even though many people claim it helps, there's no scientific evidence to back this up. If you decide to try a supplement, talk with your doctor first and expect some side effects. Men may find their breasts grow and their sex drive decreases. Saw palmetto berry extract capsules are available in most health food stores.

Fight tick paralysis with tweezers

If your fingers or toes start to tingle, then go numb; if your legs become weak and you have trouble walking; if paralysis begins to spread throughout your body, don't panic. Although you could have a serious problem, these symptoms could also be caused by a tiny bug — a tick.

Tick paralysis is a common illness in wooded parts of many countries. Here's how it happens. After a female tick mates and her eggs are fertilized, she latches onto your skin and begins to feed. As she feeds, she produces a neurotoxin that enters your bloodstream and moves throughout your body, creating havoc as it goes. The more she feeds, the more toxin she produces. Within a week, you begin to feel the paralyzing effects. Sometimes the tick will drop off by itself, and your symptoms will seem to magically go away.

And other times, she stays put, and you feel progressively worse. If you discover and remove the tick in time, your body simply flushes out the toxin, and you recover fully. But time is critical.

Because tick paralysis mimics several other conditions, particularly Guillain-Barré syndrome, a serious nerve disease, doctors spend a lot of time testing and not much time looking for ticks. If they waste too much time, you can die when the paralysis reaches your lungs.

In most tick paralysis cases, the ticks hide on your scalp. If you have long hair, they can be difficult to find. Use a fine-toothed comb, and a little patience, to rule out this easily corrected problem.

Problems with nails and hands?
It could be your hair spray

If you are having problems with your fingernails, you might need to check out your hair spray. Hair spray is a probable cause of nail disorders.

A 46-year-old woman had been using a new hair spray when she discovered some problems with her nails and hands.

Apparently, she was in the habit of spraying with one hand while running the other hand through or smoothing her hair.

She noticed that her fingernails began to "turn loose, peel and hurt." Also, the skin on the backs of her fingers began to peel.

She stopped using her hair spray and her fingers and nails both returned to normal. The distinctive ingredient in the hair spray that caused these problems is unknown.

Cosmetics are one of the most common causes of contact/irritant nail abnormalities. So, if you have "sensitive" nails and fingers and must continue to use your hair spray, try to keep the hair spray from actually touching your nails and fingers.

What your nails are trying to tell you

Can you tell how healthy you are just by looking at your nails? In some cases, you can.

Here are a few common health conditions with symptoms that can show up on the ends of your fingers.

Disease	Nail condition
Anemia	Pale nails that may become brittle, flat, or even spoon-shaped as the condition becomes more severe; long ridges can develop, also
Arthritis	Split or deformed nails
Bacterial endocarditis	A sliver-shaped hemorrhage under the nail, but without pain
Chronic infection	Clubbed fingernails (very rounded, dome-shaped nails)
Congenital heart disease	Clubbed fingernails (very rounded, dome-shaped nails)
Dermatomyositis	A sliver-shaped hemorrhage under the nail, but without pain

Disease	Nail condition
Extreme emotional stress	Bitten or chewed nails
Heart failure or chronic lung disorder	Bluish nails along with shortness of breath and a cough
Hyperthyroidism	Brittle, loose nails that are shaped like a spoon
Hypothyroidism	Brittle, loose nails
Kidney disease	White discoloration at the base of the nail
Liver disease (chronic hepatitis or cirrhosis)	Opaque, white nails
Lung cancer	Clubbed fingernails (very rounded, dome-shaped nails)
Lupus	A sliver-shaped hemorrhage under the nail, but without pain
Pituitary problems	No half-moon whiteness at the base of the nails
Psoriasis	Ends of your nails pulling away from the underlying skin (nail bed)
Recent illness or surgery	Lines or ridges that run sideways, across your nails
Trichinosis	A sliver-shaped hemorrhage under the nail, but without pain
Tuberculosis	Clubbed fingernails (very rounded, dome-shaped nails)

• •
Check your nails for cancer

Don't wait too long to see a doctor if you develop a discolored nail, either on a finger or toe. The risk is small, but there's a chance it could be cancer — and early diagnosis is critical.

Called nail-apparatus melanoma, this cancer accounts for only 1 to 2 percent of all melanomas, but it's deadly. Experts say the five-year survival rate is usually low because the cancer has spread by the time many people see a doctor.

Frequently, the only symptom is a streak running the length of your nail, from the base to the tip. Other signs, bleeding, swelling, or sores, are often mistaken for other, more common conditions. Ignoring a problem like this could be a deadly mistake.

• •

Headaches

12 ways to manage migraines naturally

Migraines can be so painful your only option is to close the curtains and stay in bed. This happens across the country 112 million times every year. If you work, it means taking a sick day, which costs employers over $13 billion in lost revenue. If you're retired, it means missing out on activities, family time, fun, and friends.

Here are some things you can try to head off a migraine disaster naturally.

Feverfew. For more than 2,000 years, feverfew has been used to treat headaches. Researchers now think they know why it works. The leaves contain chemicals that reduce the inflammation and muscle spasms associated with migraines.

In several studies, researchers gave migraine sufferers dried feverfew every day. They reported fewer and milder migraine attacks, with less vomiting. In addition, no side effects from the herb were reported. The recommended dose is 125 milligrams (mg) per day of dried feverfew leaves or two fresh leaves, chewed.

When shopping for supplements, choose products that contain at least 0.2 percent parthenolide — the main ingredient that reduces pain and the frequency of migraines. Tanetin, a flavonol in feverfew, may also fight migraines by reducing inflammation. Look for it on the label as well.

Ginger. This fragrant herb may be the root of relief for some migraine sufferers. Herbalists generally recommend 2 to 4 grams

169

of ginger a day, but for migraines, you might need more. Look for ginger root in the produce section of your supermarket or buy supplements as gelatin capsules. At first, ginger may cause a burning sensation in your mouth or stomach, so add it to your diet gradually. Make ginger tea by simmering several slices of fresh ginger root in a cup of water for about 15 minutes.

Caffeine. An over-the-counter combination of acetaminophen, aspirin, and caffeine has proven helpful for people suffering severe migraine pain. The benefits of this type of medication can last up to six hours.

Magnesium. Up to half of the people suffering from migraines don't have enough magnesium in their bodies. It's been proven that supplementing with magnesium can help reduce the number and intensity of headaches. In one study, about 80 percent of the participants reported migraine relief while taking 200 mg of magnesium a day. But remember — more isn't better. Too much magnesium can interfere with your calcium absorption. Experts recommend no more than 500 mg per day from supplements. It's a natural, inexpensive treatment without serious side effects.

Although it's easy to get magnesium from many foods in their original state, washing, peeling, and processing remove this and other important nutrients. Good food sources include brown rice, popcorn, oatmeal, cornmeal, broccoli, green peas, acorn squash, potatoes, sweet potatoes, shrimp, clams, and skim milk.

Riboflavin. One study showed daily doses of 400 mg of riboflavin, also known as vitamin B2, eases migraine pain as effectively as aspirin. If you want to get more riboflavin naturally, milk, eggs, meat, poultry, fish, and green leafy vegetables are good sources.

Fish oil. Omega-3 fish oil can reduce the number and intensity of migraines. In a study at the University of Cincinnati, 60 percent of the people reported improvement after taking fish oil capsules for six weeks. But be careful — the oil in supplements is more concentrated than in natural sources. You don't want to get too much omega-3. Your best natural source is fatty, cold-water fish, like tuna, cod, and salmon. You can also get omega-3 oil from oat germ, flaxseed, soy bean products, and walnuts.

Heat or ice. Just like any other kind of pain, you can treat migraine pain with either heat or ice. But for those who prefer a bit of cooling comfort, there are several products on the market that make it easy to grab and go. Specially shaped gel packs and pads allow you to get relief just where you need it — on your forehead, over your eyes, even on the back of your neck. These products are inexpensive, reusable, and neat.

Magnets. Using magnets for healing and pain relief is an ancient practice that's gaining popularity today. Even the National Institutes of Health considers bioelectromagnetics a true science. The most popular, and perhaps most effective, magnet therapy for migraines uses a headband with magnetized disks positioned over specific acupressure points on your head. Scientists are still unsure exactly how the magnets ease pain, but many believe it has something to do with their ability to increase blood flow. In studies, about 30 percent of migraine sufferers had moderate to substantial relief with magnet therapy.

Massage. Would you give up half an hour several times a week if it meant relief from migraine pain? Headache sufferers at the University of Miami School of Medicine did just that to receive a 30-minute head and neck massage. After five weeks, the results were impressive — fewer migraines; less painful migraines; and deeper, less interrupted sleep. Lab tests also showed much higher levels of serotonin in the group after the massages. This hormone constricts blood vessels and regulates mood and sleep.

A trained massage therapist, performing this specific routine on the back of your neck and the base of your skull, could make a huge difference in your quality of life. For a copy of the massage technique, e-mail the Touch Research Institute at field@nova.edu or call 954-262-6919.

Other alternatives. There are other alternative therapies for treating migraines that many people have tried, tested, and swear by. A psychologist associated with the Harvard Medical School and Massachusetts General Hospital in Boston combines biofeed-back, chiropractic, and acupuncture to treat migraines.

Biofeedback teaches you to control your body's automatic functions, like heart rate, blood pressure, and skin temperature. It helps people manage stress and other body functions in order to reduce migraine pain. Chiropractic decreases muscle tension that can trigger migraines. Acupuncture treats pain by targeting specific points in your body.

Even your sense of smell can ease your head pain. Studies found that people who like the smell of green apples reported less severe migraines when they sniffed this scent. Researchers aren't sure why it helps. Perhaps a pleasant smell distracts and relaxes you, lifting your mood and making it easier to handle the pain.

Talk with your doctor about trying these or other natural alternatives for your migraine pain.

• •

How to tell if it's a migraine

If you suffer from very painful headaches, it's important to find out if you have migraines. That's because migraines are treated differently than other types of headaches.

Are you sensitive to light even when you don't have a headache? That's a classic trait of people who get migraines. And with a migraine, your head pain will also react to noise and physical activity more than if you had another type of headache.

Need another clue? Almost 2,000 years ago a Greek physician suggested a quick and easy way to diagnose headaches that still works today. Sit with your head between your knees. If your head begins to pound, you have a migraine. A similar technique is to shake your head quickly from side to side. If your head pain gets worse, you have a migraine.

Although simple tests like these can help you decide if you need to take migraine medication, talk with your doctor for a professional diagnosis.

• •

Expert help for cluster headaches

At 2:00 a.m., you're suddenly jerked awake by a fierce pain on one side of your head. Your eyes may water, you may feel nauseated, your heart may beat wildly, and your blood pressure could shoot up. After about an hour, the agony goes away and you're able to sleep. But 10 minutes later, the sharp, burning pain returns. Welcome to the excruciating world of cluster headaches.

These headaches get their name from the fact that they come in bunches or "clusters." If you get one, you're likely to suffer from others within days, if not hours. They don't last long, but they do come back. Some sufferers can go for months or years without an attack, but when the clusters return, it may be for as long as two weeks of on-again, off-again torture.

The pain, which most people rate as worse than migraine pain, is sharp, stabbing, and severe. It usually affects one side of your head, but it can spread to your eyes, face, neck, and sometimes your whole head and entire upper body.

Understand the cause. Which came first, the chicken or the egg? Neurologists are asking a similar question — do cluster headaches cause brain abnormalities or do the abnormalities cause cluster headaches?

Scientists at the Institute of Neurology in London studied people suffering from cluster headaches and, using state-of-the-art technology, found permanent flaws or defects in a specific section of their brain called the hypothalamus. This area controls hunger, sex drive, and your body's natural 24-hour rhythm. Interestingly enough, this brain area shows unusual activity during a cluster headache.

This new information changes the way experts think about severe headaches, like cluster and migraine. Originally, neurologists believed your brain was healthy, but something odd happened to cause the headaches. Now, they think the brain itself is flawed. This could be the first step on the road to an effective treatment.

Avoid an attack. Although no one knows exactly what causes them, cluster headaches strike about six times more men than women. While you can't do anything about your gender, you can make some lifestyle changes that may help.

- If you're a heavy smoker or drinker, you're more likely to suffer from cluster headaches — just another reason to cut these habits out of your life.

- A higher-than-normal body temperature may be one trigger that sets off a cluster headache. Whether you are relaxing in a hot tub, sweating to the oldies, or picnicking on a summer Sunday, your body temperature is bound to rise. Within one hour, you could be suffering from a cluster headache.

- Since cluster headaches strike mostly at night, get on a regular sleep cycle. This helps your body settle more easily into deep sleep patterns.

- Avoid becoming overheated if at all possible. Sleeping in a cool bedroom may eliminate many cluster headache attacks.

Relieve the pain. Although experts don't have a sure-fire solution for cluster headaches, there are some things you can do to reduce how much they impact your life.

- Put an ice pack or cold compress against your head to lessen the pain. As with other headaches, a heating pad may work better for you — experiment to find out.

- It's an odd remedy, but try holding your hands in ice water until it becomes uncomfortable.

Even if you find ways to lessen the pain of a cluster attack, see your doctor anyway. You'll want to rule out any other problems. Also, she might be able to prescribe medication to help manage your pain.

● ●
Deadly toxin treats migraines

A bout of food poisoning can certainly give you a headache — and more. But would you believe the deadly substance that causes botulism, a severe form of food poisoning, can also bring migraine relief?

Botulinum toxin A attacks your nervous system. In severe cases, it can even paralyze your heart and lungs. Yet, it is this very action that could ease migraine pain.

In controlled studies, scientists injected the toxin into various head and facial muscles of people suffering from chronic headaches. Over time, they had less muscle pain and fewer, milder migraines. They also suffered less from nausea and noise sensitivity. Perhaps most importantly, they had no side effects.

Botulinum treatment is still experimental and quite expensive, so it may be several years before this is a common remedy for migraine sufferers.

● ●

7 super solutions for tension headaches

If you feel as if a vise is slowly squeezing your temples; if the muscles around your head, face, and neck are tense; if your whole head feels sore and pressurized, you've got a tension headache. If you get one of these headaches occasionally and can get rid of it with an over-the-counter pill, you're probably suffering from temporary stress, anxiety, fatigue, or anger. But if the pain occurs almost every day, you may be suffering from chronic tension headaches.

Here are some of the most effective natural ways to treat this pain.

Apply some pressure. The ancient Chinese art of acupressure treats many complaints caused by tension. The theory is you can press on specific points of your body to release energy blocks and relieve pain.

The following acupressure points are especially helpful at soothing tension headaches.

- Find the two small hollows on either side of your neck, just below the base of your skull. Firmly press your thumbs here — up toward your skull. Close your eyes, tilt your head back, and breathe slowly and deeply. Hold this for one to two minutes.

- With your right thumb, press into the center hollow in the back of your neck, just below the base of your skull. With your left thumb and index finger, press on either side of the bridge of your nose. For about two minutes, close your eyes, tilt your head back, and breathe deeply.

- Use the thumb of one hand to press the area between the thumb and index finger of your other hand. Make sure you apply pressure toward the base of your index finger. Hold this for about a minute, then switch hands.

For a different way to apply pressure on just the right spot, try another do-it-yourself tip. Take two tennis balls and stuff them into the toe of a nonelastic sock. Lie on your back on the carpet and place the sock under your neck with the balls just below the ridge of your skull. Soon, your tense neck and scalp muscles should relax, and your headache will slip away.

Control your aches with caffeine. Read the label on any number of pain relievers, and you'll find caffeine listed. Several years ago, researchers discovered that combining caffeine with aspirin, ibuprofen, or acetaminophen increases the effectiveness of these pain relievers — especially against tension headaches. Now, you'll find caffeine in many prescription and over-the-counter pain relievers. Just remember, they can cause side effects like dizziness, nervousness, and stomach upset.

Talk it over with a pro. If your chronic head pain is caused by depression or anxiety, you need professional help. Let your doctor determine if you have a chemical imbalance or if you need counseling. Talking with a minister, family member, or friend could also help.

Massage away tension. Because your neck and scalp muscles are involved in tension headaches, physical therapy, including massage, could be the remedy for you. It will help you stretch, strengthen, and relax your sore muscles. If you can't visit a physical therapist often, give yourself a relaxing mini-massage. Here's how:

Sit still with your eyes closed and rub your fingers over your temples and forehead or wherever you feel pain. Rub your shoulders and neck to release any tightness. Breathe slowly and deeply and concentrate on relaxing while you massage.

Treat your feet to reflexology. Who would have thought massaging your feet could relieve a tension headache. But reflexology

— the practice of using pressure on specific "zones" in your feet to relieve pain and tension in other parts of your body — can do just that.

After three months of reflexology treatments, 81 percent of people suffering from chronic tension headaches said they were cured. Of those who usually took drugs for their headache pain, 19 percent were able to stop medication completely.

Reflexology claims not only to improve circulation but to increase the amount of endorphins, natural pain relievers your body manufactures. Maybe that's why people participating in the study found they generally felt better. They said they had more energy, were able to concentrate better, were more conscious of their body and its needs, and were able to actually prevent headaches.

Stand tall. Poor posture can put a real strain on your neck muscles and contribute to annoying headaches. See if your posture passes the test. Stand with your back against a wall. Can you touch your head, heels, buttocks, and the middle of your back to the wall without straining? Can you then slide your hand between the small of your back and the wall? If you can't, or if it's difficult or painful, you need to improve your posture.

Learn to loosen up. If you get tension headaches all the time, maybe you just need to relax. No, that doesn't mean sit down and rest. It means you need deep, internal relaxation involving your muscles, your breathing, and your mind. With formal training, you'll learn how to "read" your body — when do you feel stress, when do your muscles tighten up, when do you clench your teeth — and you'll learn how to control the way your body responds to stress.

● ●

Watch out for secret stroke risk

If you're young, you probably don't think about suffering a stroke. But in some cases, youth is no protection against this killer.

Many migraine sufferers are familiar with the added agony of auras — stabbing or flashing light during a migraine that can make the simplest activity a nightmare. Now scientists are saying there may be a link between migraine auras and strokes, no matter what your age.

Almost half of all people experiencing migraines plus auras may also suffer from a dangerous heart condition — one that could allow blood clots to flow directly into the brain. This condition, called patent foramen ovale, means you are a prime candidate for a stroke. In fact, an Italian study found that having migraines with auras was the only risk factor for the women under 35 who had suffered a stroke.

Here's the evidence of a connection between migraines and stroke:

- Many people report their strokes occur during a typical migraine attack. Severe headaches occur in 25 percent of strokes.

- Researchers found that during the aura phase of young migraine sufferers, blood flow to the brain was severely restricted — almost reaching stroke-causing levels.

- Many people suffering from migraines also have blood that's more likely to clot. This could be due to a defect in the cells lining the heart and blood vessels.

If you are a young woman who has migraines plus auras, most doctors will tell you not to smoke or take birth control pills — two factors that will raise your risk of stroke even higher. And anyone with migraines plus auras should see a heart specialist.

● ●

Fast fixes for sinus headaches

A sinus headache can cause unbearable pain and pressure around your eyes and in your cheeks. If you need relief, try these proven tips.

- Use a vaporizer. The warm, moist air will help your sinuses drain.

- Drink eight to 10 glasses of fluid a day to thin the mucus and clear your nasal passages.

- Put extra pillows under your head when you sleep so mucus won't drain back into your sinuses. If sinus pressure is worse on one side, sleep on the other side.

- Take a hot shower. The steam will help clear your nasal passages and relieve the pain and pressure.

- Eating hot, spicy foods or herbs, such as hot chilies, horseradish, or garlic, will help open your nasal passages.

- A nasal wash using warm salt water and a rubber syringe can be a huge help in treating and preventing sinusitis.

- An over-the-counter nasal spray can give you relief, but don't use it longer than three days. Instead, ask your doctor to prescribe a corticosteroid spray to reduce inflammation in your nose.

- Place a washcloth soaked in warm water on your face — over your nose, cheeks, and forehead. The moist heat should bring some relief.

- Pinpoint and eliminate the cause. Your sinus headache could be caused by hay fever or some other allergen in your environment. Keep track of when and where your headaches strike.

- If the discharge from your stuffy nose turns greenish-yellow, it's time to see your doctor. You could have a sinus infection.

●●●●●●●●●●●●●●●●●●●●●●●●●●●●

Heal the hurt with herbs

Ginkgo helps relieve headaches and halt confusion by increasing blood flow to the brain — by as much as 70 percent in seniors. And it seems the longer you take ginkgo, the more it helps. Although it has no known serious side effects, very large doses may cause restlessness, diarrhea, nausea, or vomiting.

Rosemary, lavender, and chamomile are essential oils that may help ease your headache. For quick comfort, gently rub just one drop onto your skin where it hurts the most.

And believe it or not, an herbal footbath might soak your headache pain away. In a big plastic basin, mix one teaspoon of powdered mustard or ginger with water as hot as you can stand. Settle into a comfortable chair, ease both feet gently into the water, and drape a thick towel across the basin to hold in the heat. Lean back, close your eyes, breathe deeply, and relax for about 15 minutes. By the time the water cools, your headache should be gone.

Scientists studying aromatherapy say that simply smelling peppermint will relax your muscles and help you think and concentrate better. Now there's more scientific proof peppermint oil is as effective as acetaminophen in reducing headache pain.

A solution of peppermint oil, eucalyptus oil, and ordinary alcohol will soothe your nerves, relax the muscles in your head and neck, and ease your pain. Simply sponge it on your forehead and temples.

●●●●●●●●●●●●●●●●●●●●●●●●

Hidden causes of headache pain

Apart from the four main types of headaches — sinus, tension, migraine, and cluster — you may suffer head pain from alcohol, acute glaucoma, certain types of arthritis, and several other causes.

Hunger. If you skip a meal, hunger can really cause a pain in your brain. This ache is your body's way of telling you to stop what you are doing and eat. Grab a piece of fruit or some vegetables, or sit down to a high-carbohydrate meal, like pasta. If you need something really fast, try a glass of orange juice. It will give you quick energy.

Drug side effect. It's quite common to develop a headache as a side effect of any medication. If you think a drug could be causing your pounding head, talk with your doctor. He might need to change your prescription or lower your dose. Be sure you always take the prescribed amount at the recommended time. Changing your dose or schedule can cause headaches. Read the label and package insert carefully for any over-the-counter drugs you use. If you're taking more than one medication, your headache might be caused by a drug interaction. Avoid drinking alcohol when you are taking medicine. This combination can bring on headaches and other, more serious, side effects. Illegal or recreational drugs can cause headaches, coma, and death.

Heat. High temperatures and direct sun are the perfect recipe for a heat headache. The best solution for this kind of pain is to get out of the sun and bring your body temperature down to normal. Drink cool, not cold, liquids and sit in front of a gentle fan. If you go back out into the sun, put on a wide-brimmed hat to keep the rays off your head. Wear lightweight, light-colored, loose clothing to help you stay cool. If possible, take breaks and drink plenty of liquids to keep your body from becoming overheated.

Teeth grinding. Grinding your teeth while you sleep is another sneaky cause of daytime headaches. If you suspect this might be the source of your pain, have your dentist check your pearly whites for signs of grinding. And avoid chewing gum for a while to give your jaw a rest.

High blood pressure. This headache is easy to avoid — simply keep your blood pressure under control. To do this, learn to manage stressful situations. Relieve anxiety by exercising, breathing deeply, listening to restful music, or meditating. Take your blood pressure medication as your doctor instructed — never skip a dose. And if you are overweight, lose a few pounds.

Giant cell arteritis. A particularly bad or unusual headache can be a sign of real trouble for people over 55. Giant cell arteritis is a disease that inflames your blood vessels and produces severe head pain. If your other symptoms include muscle pain in your shoulders and hips, sweating, fever, jaw pain when chewing, and loss of appetite, see your doctor right away. If you test positive for giant cell arteritis, you'll need immediate treatment to prevent blindness.

Heart disease

Getting 'steamed' can fry your heart

Do you know someone who has an irritating tendency to interrupt you in the middle of a sentence? If so, that person may be more likely to develop heart disease than most people. But, by the same token, if you feel angry when you get interrupted, you may also be at increased risk for heart disease. A recent study found that having a dominant personality, which is characterized by interrupting people or being easily irritated, is a risk factor for heart disease.

Anger and its associated emotions have long been associated with heart attack. For example, one recent study found that people who scored high on a hostility scale were more likely to be insulin resistant, overweight, and carry their extra weight in the upper body — all risk factors for heart disease.

Another study suggests that a mental stress test might be more effective than a physical stress test in predicting who will get heart disease. Researchers found that people who reported high levels of irritability during mental tests designed to measure frustration were more likely to have ischemia, a reduced supply of oxygen to the heart.

Since most people these days spend more time under mental stress, rather than physical stress, finding ways to cope with anger and frustration could be one of the best ways to protect yourself from heart disease. Here are some steps to take as soon as you feel your anger rising.

Breathe deeply. Taking a few deep breaths will help you calm down and relax. You'll also be sending much-needed oxygen to your racing heart. That old saying about counting to 10 is good advice, too. Just count slowly and think calm thoughts.

Express it — then forget it. Holding anger in can be even more damaging than expressing it. However, if you express your anger, do so in a constructive way. Wait until you are calm and can say what you need to without exploding. State clearly why you are angry, but try not to accuse others if you can help it. You might be able to bring about positive change in a situation. But even if nothing changes, express yourself — then let it go.

Find a sympathetic ear. Talking with a loved one or close friend about an issue that is angering you will usually help you get a clearer perspective. Ask someone who isn't as involved to help you come up with a good plan of attack to solve the problem.

Give the other guy a break. A little competition can be healthy, but some people never stop competing. They always have to be first in line, pass everyone on the highway — always the winner. But all that anger and stress can hurt your heart, making you the loser. Try letting go and letting the other guy win sometimes.

The following steps for coping with anger are the ones to take over the long haul. Even though you may not get immediate results, stick with them, and you should see dramatic improvements in your ability to handle anger.

Exercise. A long walk in pleasant surroundings or working up a sweat in your garden may be just the thing to help you replace bad feelings with good ones. Along with strengthening your heart and lowering your blood pressure, regular exercise reduces stress and gives you a feeling of well-being.

Lend a helping hand. No matter how bad you think your situation is, you can always find someone with more problems. If you're angry much of the time, it's probably because you are focusing on yourself and your feelings. Try doing some volunteer work or helping a neighbor or friend. Giving of yourself helps you get a better focus on the rest of the world.

Escape. Sometimes a short "mental vacation" is just what you need to give you some distance from the stressful situation. Read a book, watch a pleasant movie, or lose yourself in your favorite hobby. Then you can go back to working on the problem with a calmer attitude.

Learn stress management. Learning stress management techniques can help you put your life in better perspective. Instead of getting angry about the countless little things that can go wrong in a day, choose to let go of them so anger never arises at all. Save your anger for the things that really matter and use it to spur you into action.

Avoid the issue. Perhaps the smartest way to deal with anger is to avoid the situations you know will cause it. If shopping in crowded stores infuriates you, shop on Tuesday nights when fewer people are out, instead of on Saturdays or the day after Thanksgiving. If traffic makes you crazy, arrange to go in to work earlier or later than the rush hour, and leave at an off time, too. If discussing politics with your brother-in-law always leads to a heated argument, don't be drawn into a conversation.

You can choose to live a calmer, happier life. And one of the biggest benefits is a healthier heart.

Early warnings of heart disease

In the movies, you know a man is having a heart attack when he clutches his chest and slumps over. In real life, you may get warning signals long before you have a heart attack.

A recent study found a connection between hair growth in men under 60 years of age and heart disease. Baldness and having a hairy chest, which often occur together, were associated with an increased risk of heart disease.

The same study found that having a diagonal crease in your earlobe was also associated with an increase in heart disease risk.

You may not be able to do anything about your bald head or your hairy chest, but they could be giving you a warning — take good care of your heart.

• •

Simple changes in lifestyle — clean living and clean diet — can reverse heart disease

You know the old saying, "The more things change, the more they stay the same." Well, in the case of heart disease, the saying could go something like this: "The more things change, the more they go back to the way they were."

Making changes in your lifestyle can help your heart and blood vessels go back to how they were before your doctor told you that you have heart disease.

Following a low-fat vegetarian diet, clean living and stress management can reverse heart disease in many people in as little as a year, some scientists are saying.

In a one-year experiment, 41 volunteers (men and women ages 35 to 75) agreed to make some lifestyle changes to help reverse their existing heart disease.

An experimental group of 22 volunteers agreed to a substantial change in their habits: They ate a low-fat vegetarian diet, exercised regularly and went to a stress management class.

They also didn't smoke or drink caffeine, and the amount of alcohol that they drank was limited to two drinks a day. The 19 volunteers in the control group stuck to a program that is usually recommended by doctors for heart patients: They didn't smoke, did moderate exercise and limited their dietary fat to 30 percent of total calories.

At the end of the study, 18 of the 22 volunteers who made substantial lifestyle changes showed reversal of their heart disease.

The arteries that had been clogged were clean. The blood vessels started looking as clean and clear as they had before they developed heart disease.

The people in this experimental group reduced their angina (chest pain) frequency by 91 percent, their angina duration, 42 percent, and their angina severity, 28 percent. The study also indicated that the sickest people made the greatest improvements, and those improvements seemed to occur more readily in women.

Out of the group of 19 volunteers who followed the usual moderate medical advice, only eight showed any improvement. Ten others actually got worse. Their angina frequency, duration and severity all increased.

The changes and reversal of heart disease in the volunteers in the substantial-lifestyle-change group are similar to the changes doctors expect to see with cholesterol-lowering drugs.

But these people achieved their results with sensible changes in diet, stress management and exercise habits without having to depend on drugs.

Although eight of the people in the usual-care group got better, the study suggests that we should fight against heart disease more aggressively.

Microscopic menace may infect arteries

Scientists are finding more and more evidence that a bacterial infection could cause heart disease. This would explain the cycle of heart disease occurrences from 1940 to 1970. Scientists say the rise and fall in numbers is strangely similar to that of an infectious epidemic.

Researchers are investigating the theory that *Chlamydia pneumoniae*, bacteria that cause sinusitis, bronchitis, and pneumonia, may also damage arterial walls. This damage eventually leads to a buildup of cholesterol or an increase in blood clots, both risk factors for heart disease.

Scientists took notice of this theory when they were studying a group of people suffering from atherosclerosis. They found that more than 73 percent had *C. pneumoniae* in the arteries of their hearts. Only 4 percent of the group without atherosclerosis had evidence of the bacteria.

Now, researchers studying Alaska Natives have found that *C. pneumoniae* were present in plaques found in the arteries of 60 people who died in accidents. The interesting news for researchers was that the bacteria were also present in blood samples of 56 of those 60 people up to 26 years before their deaths.

Before a substance can be established as a cause of a disease, it has to be proven to be present before the disease is diagnosed. This new study supports the theory that the presence of *C. pneumoniae* in clogged arteries is more than a coincidence — which could lead to new ways to prevent and treat heart and artery disease.

Tiny pill packs powerful protection

Open your medicine cabinet, and you'll probably see the answer to a longer life — if you're at risk of a heart attack. Over 80 billion aspirin are taken by Americans each year for aches, pains, and headaches, and it's the main ingredient in more than 50 over-the-counter products.

Aspirin therapy has also become the "gold standard" for treating people who have suffered a heart attack or are at risk of one. Salicylic acid, the main ingredient in aspirin, keeps blood cells from clumping together and sticking to the walls of your arteries. This reduces your risk of blood clots and heart attacks.

Aspirin therapy involves taking small doses, one 81-milligram (mg) baby aspirin, every day to help keep your blood free of clots. However, the latest research says a larger, booster dose — about 325 mg or one regular aspirin — twice a month might be necessary for aspirin therapy to maintain its effectiveness. After about two weeks, that dose wears off and another one is needed. Experts recommend a 325-mg dose on the 1st and 15th of each month and a smaller, 81-mg dose the rest of the month.

If you are a man over 40 or a woman over 50 with any heart disease risk factors, like high blood pressure, high cholesterol, diabetes, a family history of early heart attack, or if you are a smoker or postmenopausal woman not taking hormones, aspirin therapy might be beneficial for you.

In 1997, the FDA approved a prescription blood-thinner, clopidogrel, for treating and preventing heart disease. But a recent study, taking into account cost, convenience, and safety, found that aspirin is still the best choice for most people. Yet, the study found that clopidogrel may be a better choice for people with peripheral arterial disease. This disease causes the arteries outside your heart, like those that deliver blood to your arms and legs, to become clogged. It may also be an option for people who have severe side effects from aspirin therapy.

Always talk to your doctor before beginning aspirin therapy on your own to be sure it's the best choice for you. If you're taking ACE inhibitors for congestive heart failure, for example, aspirin may do more harm than good. A recent study found that when aspirin was given to people taking ACE inhibitors, certain aspects of lung function became worse.

● ●
Pine-bark extract alternative to aspirin

If your doctor recommends aspirin therapy but aspirin bothers your stomach, here's good news. A nutritional supplement called Pycnogenol may be a good alternative, especially if you're a smoker.

A recent study found that Pycnogenol, which is made from a certain type of pine tree found only in France, may work like aspirin to reduce the "stickiness" of blood cells.

Smoking and stress can trigger the release of adrenaline, a stress hormone, which causes platelets in your blood to become stickier. This can lead to the formation of blood clots that could cause a heart attack or stroke.

Researchers gave smokers aspirin or Pycnogenol, and then tested their blood two hours after they had smoked a cigarette. Both aspirin and Pycnogenol reduced smoke-induced platelet stickiness, but Pycnogenol did not increase bleeding time, like aspirin. And here's another benefit — a smaller dose was required to achieve the same effects.

You can find Pycnogenol at most health food stores, but check with your doctor before taking any supplement, especially if you have heart disease, or if you're taking any medication.

● ●

Eat hearty food for a healthy heart

If you want a healthy heart, feed it healthy food. You know you should avoid foods high in saturated fats and cholesterol, but do you know what foods you should eat? Here are four of the best foods for heart health.

Whole grains. One of the best and easiest ways to improve your health is to eat more fiber. Just trading in your bacon and egg breakfast for a bowl of cereal every morning could save your life someday.

One long-term study of more than 40,000 male health professionals tracked their eating habits over a six-year period. Researchers found that the risk of a fatal heart attack was 55 percent lower for the men who ate the most fiber. Most of these men started their day off with a bowl of cold breakfast cereal.

The researchers concluded that you could cut your risk of heart attack by 20 percent just by adding 10 grams of fiber a day to your diet. That's the same impact you would get by lowering your cholesterol by 10 percent.

Women reap heart-healthy benefits from a high-fiber diet, too. One study found that women who ate the most whole-grain products lowered their risk of heart disease by more than 30 percent compared with women who ate the least amount. Researchers think whole-grain foods may play a role in lowering heart disease risk by improving the way your body uses insulin.

Adding fiber doesn't have to be boring. The women in the study ate popcorn, oatmeal, whole-grain breakfast cereal, wheat germ, brown rice, bran, dark bread, and other grains.

Soy. The Food and Drug Administration (FDA) allows soy products to carry a label advertising the heart benefits of soy. That should tell you how strong the evidence is — especially if you're also eating low fat.

One recent study compared a regular low-fat diet with a low-fat diet that also doubled intake of soluble fiber and replaced most animal protein with vegetable protein from soy. Compared with the regular low-fat diet, the one containing soy protein significantly lowered total cholesterol levels and bad LDL cholesterol, but it didn't reduce the levels of good HDL cholesterol.

Try using soy flour or soy milk in your baking, or add a little tofu to your salad. But don't just add soy products to a typical American diet. Most Americans eat too much protein already, and if you add protein-rich soybeans to a meat-heavy diet, you're likely to have kidney trouble. Your kidneys will have to work overtime to excrete all the waste that is produced when your body metabolizes protein.

(New research claims soy may accelerate brain aging. For more information, see the Mental impairment chapter.)

Vegetables. You know you should eat your veggies. They're low in calories, high in fiber, most contain no fat, and they're loaded with nutrients. You may not know that most vegetables also contain compounds known as lignins. A recent study found that men with high blood levels of a lignin called enterolactone had three times less heart disease than men with low levels. Good sources of enterolactone include seed oils, particularly flaxseed oil, whole grain cereals, seaweeds, and beans.

Fish. A tasty salmon steak for dinner or tuna for lunch once a week can help protect your heart and arteries. Fatty fish like salmon, tuna, sardines, herring, and mackerel contain omega-3 fatty acids. Omega 3s help keep your blood from becoming too sticky and forming clots, which can cause heart attack and stroke. Fish oil also lowers your bad cholesterol and triglyceride levels, and it helps protect against irregular heartbeats.

Studies show that eating just one 3-ounce serving of fatty fish per week can cut your risk of heart attack in half. And a recent study found that taking a daily fish oil supplement reduced risk of death, stroke, or another heart attack by 10 percent in people who had already had a heart attack.

If you include even a moderate amount of fish in your diet, you can lower your risk of heart disease by 50 to 70 percent. So dish up some fish and do your heart some good.

Refreshing juice zaps heart disease

The next time you order a hamburger at a drive-through restaurant, be kind to your heart and drink a glass of apple juice with it instead of soda.

Apple juice is a new heavyweight contender in the fight against heart disease. It joins tea, red wine, and grape juice as an antioxidant-rich drink.

Previous research found that red wine protected against heart disease. Then researchers discovered that flavonoids, chemicals found naturally in grape skins and other foods, were responsible for the heart-healthy benefits of red wine. This also explained why red wine was beneficial and white wine wasn't. The grape skins are removed during the production of white wine.

And a recent study found that purple grape juice produced the same beneficial effects as red wine, regardless of alcohol content — good news for teetotalers.

Now a new study shows that grape juice isn't the only heart-protective fruit juice. Apple juice is more nutritious than previously thought.

Researchers tested six brands of commercial, no sugar added apple juice. They also tested the flesh and peel of fresh apples, as well as whole Red Delicious apples. Although the apples and juice contained varying amounts of flavonoids, they all prevented bad LDL cholesterol from becoming oxidized.

An earlier Dutch study tested 805 men over the age of 65 to see what effect their intake of foods containing flavonoids had on their risk of heart disease. Men who consumed the most flavonoids in the form of apples, tea, and onions had a significantly lower risk of heart disease than those who didn't consume foods high in flavonoids. A follow-up study in Finland reinforced these results.

Besides being a good source of antioxidants, apples provide the soluble fiber pectin, which seems to bind LDL cholesterol and help it move out of your body. Apples also contain healthy amounts of vitamins C and E.

For a refreshing way to help keep your arteries clear and your heart pumping strong, drink some apple or grape juice every day.

Words you need to know

Angina pectoris — pain in the chest, arms, or jaw caused by lack of oxygen to the heart

Antioxidants — substances that protect cells from damage by neutralizing free radicals

Arteriosclerosis — hardening of the arteries

Atherosclerosis — narrowing of the arteries due to the deposits of fat and other substances

Cholesterol — a substance in your body that plays a role in the transport of fats in your bloodstream

Coronary heart disease — any disorder that restricts the blood supply to the heart

Free radicals — unstable molecules that can damage cells

Congestive heart failure — when the heart is unable to pump blood well enough to maintain good circulation

High-density lipoprotein (HDL) — known as "good" cholesterol because it carries cholesterol away from the arteries to the liver, where it is broken down and disposed of

Hypercholesterolemia — high level of blood cholesterol resulting from an inherited disorder or a high-fat diet

Hypertension — high blood pressure

Lipoproteins — substances in your blood that are made up of lipids (fats) and proteins

Low-density lipoprotein (LDL) — also known as "bad" cholesterol because high levels can build up on the walls of your arteries and combine with other substances to form a hard deposit called plaque

Myocardial infarction — when an area of the heart muscle dies because it was deprived of its blood supply, also known as a heart attack

● ●

Brew some tea for your heart's sake

Tea is the most common beverage in the world — next to water. And a spot of green or black tea might be just the thing if you want to keep your heart and arteries in good shape.

Tea contains flavonoids, which act as powerful antioxidants that keep cholesterol from damaging artery walls. The flavonoids found in green tea, called catechins, are especially effective.

A recent study found that people who drank three cups of tea daily for six weeks had increased levels of antioxidants in their blood. Research shows that tea may protect against heart disease in other ways, too.

Builds better arteries. If you want your arteries to remain strong and free of clogs, a cup of tea may help. In a recent study, volunteers drank about three cups of black tea every day. After four weeks, their arteries resisted the build up of cholesterol. Another study found that the more tea people drank, the less likely they were to have atherosclerosis, a buildup of plaque in the arteries.

Lowers cholesterol. High cholesterol increases your risk of heart disease, but regular tea consumption may help keep cholesterol under control. One Japanese study that followed tea drinkers over the course of nearly five years showed that having several cups of green tea a day reduced cholesterol and triglyceride levels significantly.

Helps control weight. New research suggests that green tea could also help reduce your risk of heart disease by helping to control your weight.

In one study, young men took two capsules of green tea extract plus caffeine, caffeine alone, or a placebo at each meal for six weeks. The men who took the green tea capsules burned more calories in a 24-hour period than the other men. There was no difference between the caffeine-only group and the placebo group.

If further studies support this finding, green tea could be a healthy addition to a sensible weight loss program. And unlike caffeine and ephedra, another common ingredient in weight-loss supplements, green tea doesn't raise heart rate and blood pressure.

Drinking tea won't compensate for an unhealthy lifestyle, but relaxing with a cup of tea is an easy, enjoyable way to keep your heart healthy.

A nutty way to help your heart

The evidence is piling up — nuts are good for your heart. Although they are high in fat, they are low in saturated fat and cholesterol free. Most nuts are a rich source of monounsaturated fatty acids (MUFAs), the same kind found in olive oil, or polyunsaturated fatty acids (PUFAs), which are also found in fish oil.

Researchers studying 30,000 Seventh Day Adventists found that those who ate nuts at least five times a week reduced their risk of heart attack by 50 percent, compared with those who ate them less than once a week.

What kind of nuts do you like? If you don't overdo it, you can enjoy your favorite nuts without gaining weight and make your heart healthier to boot.

Walnuts. One study of people living in a walnut-producing area of France found that a high intake of walnuts was associated with an increase in good HDL cholesterol. Walnuts also increased a substance called apo A1, which is associated with a lower risk of heart disease.

Peanuts. Technically, peanuts aren't nuts — they're legumes. Yet, they may provide a unique way to get heart-healthy MUFAs. Peanuts contain the same antioxidant found in grape skins, and this antioxidant is partly responsible for red wine's ability to lower heart disease risk.

One study tested five different kinds of diets — a typical American diet, a low-fat diet, an olive-oil diet, a peanut/peanut butter diet, and a peanut oil diet. The peanut diets contained small amounts of peanuts daily. The study found that the olive oil and the peanut diets, which were low in saturated fat and high in monounsaturated fat, all lowered bad LDL cholesterol. The low-fat diet lowered bad LDL cholesterol, too, but it also lowered good HDL cholesterol and raised triglyceride levels.

Almonds. Scientists recently tested the cholesterol-lowering effects of adding almonds to the diet. Thirty men and women (ages 29 to 81) enrolled in a study at the YMCA Cardiac Rehabilitation Unit in Palo Alto, California.

The men and women in the study stayed on a low-in-saturated-fats diet for nine weeks. During that time, they ate 100 grams of almonds a day (50 grams as whole raw almonds, and 50 grams as ground almonds). That's the equivalent of almost four ounces per day of almonds. Each person kept a food diary, and the scientists took measurements of blood-cholesterol levels throughout the nine weeks.

At the end of the nine weeks, the investigators reported that the average total cholesterol level of 235 was reduced by about 20 points. The nearly 9-percent reduction in the total cholesterol level was due to a reduction in the level of LDL cholesterol in the blood (the "bad cholesterol"). Scientists explained that the almonds weren't fat-free. But, they contain monounsaturated fats (the good fat).

The increase in monounsaturated fats (almonds) and the decrease in saturated fats helped lower blood-cholesterol levels.

Chocolate lovers live longer

If you feel guilty every time you sneak a candy bar, take heart — especially if your candy of choice is chocolate. According to research, you can indulge your sweet tooth, within reason, with a clear conscience.

Researchers at Harvard Medical School found that men who ate candy lived, on average, about a year longer than men who didn't eat candy. Good news — considering Americans eat an average of 14 pounds of chocolate and almost 12 pounds of other candy yearly.

While this study didn't differentiate between chocolate and other types of candy, researchers theorized that antioxidant phenols in chocolate could be responsible for the life-prolonging effect. A one-and-a-half ounce piece of chocolate contains as much phenol as a glass of red wine — and a moderate intake of red wine is known to protect against heart disease.

Another study found that healthy people who drank a tablespoon of cocoa powder in water took longer to form blood clots, apparently because the cocoa slowed down the clotting action of platelets. This could reduce heart attack and stroke risk the same way a daily aspirin does.

And a recent study found that chocolate increases sex drive in women. While this might not have anything to do with health or longevity, men may be encouraged to know that all those heart-shaped boxes of chocolates at Valentine's Day do serve a purpose.

All this adds up to the fact that chocolate isn't so bad after all, and it may even be good for you. As usual, moderation is the key. Too much of almost anything is bad for you, and too much chocolate can pack on some decidedly unhealthy pounds.

If you're a victim of irresistible chocolate cravings, experts offer some advice — don't eat chocolate when you're hungry. A recent study found that chocolate cravers who waited until 15 minutes after a meal to indulge their chocolate urge reduced their craving to the level of noncravers. Researchers say you learn to crave chocolate if you regularly use it to satisfy your hunger.

So don't overdo it, and you can savor your chocolate with the knowledge that you might be improving your health.

Get moving for a healthier heart

One of the best things you can do for your heart is to keep your body moving. Unfortunately, most people don't get enough exercise. That's one of the reasons heart disease is the number one killer today. Here are some ways exercise keeps your heart in good shape.

Lowers blood pressure. New evidence shows that physical activity lowers blood pressure, even without weight loss. And, according to a new study, lower blood pressure persists even after exercise. The study found that blood pressure was significantly lower for up to 16 hours after one 45-minute exercise session. So even if your exercise efforts don't yield a smaller waistline, don't give up. Your heart is still reaping great benefits.

Controls cholesterol. Exercise lowers cholesterol, too. One study on postmenopausal women found that exercise reduced cholesterol levels almost three times as much as a similar reduction in calorie intake. Yet, consistency in exercise may be the key to reducing cholesterol. In a study of a group of men, regular exercise decreased the risk of oxidation of bad LDL cholesterol, but short bursts of exercise actually seemed to increase the risk, as well as increasing the risk of plaque formation in blood vessels.

You don't have to become a muscleman or run a marathon to get heart-healthy benefits from exercise. Any activity is better than none. One study found that people who exercised just 30 minutes to two hours a week had reductions in blood pressure, resting heart rate, and body mass index — and all of these things can improve heart health.

What kind of exercise is best for you? Simply walking may be the best and least expensive way to lower your heart disease risk. According to one study, walking at least 10 blocks a day was associated with a 33 percent lower risk of heart attack.

And if you really can't seem to fit time into your day to take a walk or do other exercise, don't be discouraged. Research shows that incorporating physical activity into daily life can work as well as a structured exercise program. Two recent studies compared the effects of an exercise program with lifestyle changes, like taking the stairs instead of the elevator. The studies showed similar reductions in blood pressure and total and LDL cholesterol in both the structured exercise group and the lifestyle changes group.

Here's the moral of the story — to keep your heart healthy, do whatever you can to keep your body moving.

Help your heart keep a steady beat

Your heart usually beats steady as a clock, but every once in a while, you may feel a quick fluttering. It's as if your heart "skips a beat." This irregularity is called arrhythmia, and most of the time, it's nothing to worry about. It happens to everyone, and as you age, you're more likely to experience arrhythmias.

Some arrhythmias are caused by stress, tobacco, caffeine, alcohol, or certain medications, while others are a symptom of heart disease. Sometimes, the arrhythmias themselves can be dangerous.

When your heart beats too slowly, it is called bradycardia. With this condition, your heart may slow down too much and just stop beating. It may be a symptom of an underlying disease, or it could mean your heart medication, such as a beta blocker, is slowing your heartbeat too much.

When your heartbeat is too fast, it's called tachycardia. This can be caused by stress, too much caffeine, or certain types of medication, especially diet pills. While everyone's heartbeat speeds up occasionally, if you have episodes of tachycardia often, or if the episodes last longer than a few minutes, see your doctor. If your tachycardia continues for an extended time, it could lead to congestive heart failure or heart attack.

If you have an irregular heartbeat, your doctor might prescribe medicine to help, but here are some other things you can do.

- **Exercise.** Regular exercise is the best way to prevent arrhythmias. The healthier and stronger your heart is, the better it can maintain its own rhythm. Check with your doctor to see what kind of exercise she recommends for you.

- **Lessen stress.** If you have a problem with arrhythmia, it's even more important for you to find ways to deal with stress. Studies show there is an increase in the number of sudden deaths during natural disasters, like earthquakes. A new study suggests stress might trigger dangerous arrhythmias. Researchers studied people with ventricular arrhythmia, a type of arrhythmia that can be life threatening. When the people were put under stress — by taking a math test or being reminded of a bad memory — they were more likely to experience an abnormally fast heart rate.

- **Don't smoke.** Aside from its other health risks, smoking makes your heart beat faster and your blood vessels narrow. This could make smoking a big contributor to tachycardia. Many products and programs are available to help you quit smoking. Choose one and stop.

- **Dodge diet pills.** The amphetamines and other stimulants in many diet pills, whether prescription or over-the-counter, can trigger tachycardia. A slow, steady weight loss program is a better approach to solving a weight problem.

- **Cut down on caffeine.** You may think of your morning cup of coffee as a pleasant ritual, but it may not be the best thing for your heart. Caffeine stimulates your heart and can cause palpitations and tachycardia. If rapid heartbeat is a problem for you, it's better to stay away from the caffeine in coffee, tea, and cola drinks.

- **Beware of drug interactions.** Tell your doctor about any drugs you are taking, including over-the-counter drugs, when she prescribes a new one. Drug interactions can cause tachycardia. And learn to read labels carefully. Some ingredients in decongestants and other medicines may cause an irregular heartbeat.

- **Don't let depression keep you down.** A recent study shows that depressed people have as much as 30 percent more of a hormone called norepinephrine in their blood than people who aren't depressed. Norepinephrine raises your heart rate, so you don't want too much of it in your body. If you're depressed, get counseling.

• •
Simple relief for a racing heart

Here's a natural way to slow your racing heart. Get a big bowl of ice water, hold your breath, and dunk your face. This technique is often enough of a shock to restore your normal heartbeat. A big bag of ice cubes or a towel dipped in ice water, held over your face for just a moment, may work as well.

A word of caution — if you have angina or chest pain that gets worse in cold weather, don't try this home remedy. Call your doctor.
• •

4 drug-free ways to triumph over heart disease

Heart disease is a killer, and the best way to avoid being a victim is to practice prevention. If you already have heart disease or high blood pressure, or even if you've had heart surgery, you still have the power to increase your odds of beating this disease. And the most powerful weapons you have might be your mind, your church, and your family.

Optimism. If you have heart problems, look on the bright side — it could help you live longer. According to research, a positive attitude can increase your chances of surviving heart problems. Studies find that people with a positive attitude, high self-esteem, and a sense of control over their lives do better after a heart attack.

One study on people who had undergone angioplasty found that those who scored low on measures of self-esteem, optimism, and being in control of their lives were two and a half times more likely to have a heart attack or require another angioplasty or bypass surgery.

A similar study followed people who had undergone heart bypass surgery for six months after the surgery. Researchers found that the most optimistic people were 50 percent less likely to be hospitalized again for subsequent heart problems, like infection, angina, or a second operation to reopen clogged arteries.

And an optimistic attitude may help you live longer, even if you don't have heart problems. One 30-year study found that people who scored high on the pessimistic end of a personality test had a 19 percent greater risk of dying than people who scored high on optimism.

Meditation. Your doctor can give you medicine to help lower your blood pressure, but about half of the people stop taking their medicine after one year, usually because of unpleasant side effects. Proper diet and exercise will also help lower blood pressure, but many people find it difficult to follow that advice.

Another way to lower your blood pressure is to practice meditation. Meditation helps you relax, and it opens up your blood vessels, making it easier for your heart to pump blood throughout your body. Find an instructor who can teach you proper meditation techniques, and you might be able to lower your blood pressure without medication.

One study on African-Americans with high blood pressure showed that those who practiced meditation for three months reduced their systolic blood pressure (the top number) an average of 10 to 12 points and their diastolic blood pressure (the bottom number) six to eight points. These reductions are similar to those achieved by taking blood pressure medication. But remember — follow your doctor's advice. Don't stop taking your medication without his approval.

Prayer. When you're in distress, saying a prayer can make you feel better — but that's not all. Researchers found incredible evidence that people who are prayed for benefit, even when they don't realize they're being prayed for.

In one study, the first names of heart patients were given to a group of people from various religions who prayed for them daily for four weeks. The patients never met the people who were praying for them, and they weren't even aware that anyone was praying for them. Nevertheless, researchers found an 11-percent reduction in scores of heart disease severity in the prayer group compared with a group that wasn't prayed for.

Family support. Numerous studies have found that strong social support can lower your risk of disease. People with heart disease may especially benefit from a supportive family.

A recent study found that married people with supportive relationships respond better to stress than couples with a low level of social support. Researchers studied 45 couples and measured their blood pressure and other responses to stress. Men with supportive relationships showed a lower increase in blood pressure, as well as less constriction of their blood vessels. Women with supportive relationships had less constriction of blood vessels, but the increase in blood pressure was about the same. Researchers say these improvements in stress response translate into less stress on your heart.

●●●●●●●●●●●●●●●●●●●●●●●●●
Bypass surgery warning

A recent study found that people who become depressed after having coronary artery bypass surgery are three times more likely to experience heart failure, heart attack, or other heart problem in the first year after their surgery.

About 20 percent of the people who have bypass surgery become depressed while still in the hospital. If you're one of them, don't hesitate to tell your doctor. Treating your depression may save your life.

●●●●●●●●●●●●●●●●●●●●●●●

Heartburn

15 ways to cool the heat of heartburn

Heartburn is spreading like wildfire. Almost 25 million people experience that uncomfortable burning sensation in their chests every day, and more than one out of three people have heartburn at least once a month. Unfortunately, according to a recent study, most people don't know the risk factors for heartburn or what they can do to prevent it.

Heartburn is the most common symptom of gastroesophageal reflux disease (GERD). While GERD isn't a life-threatening condition, it is unpleasant and can sometimes cause digestive complications, like erosion of your esophagus and teeth.

Heartburn occurs when stomach acid flows back up your esophagus, the tube that carries food to your stomach. It can be triggered by certain foods or beverages. Lifestyle factors, such as stress, cigarette smoking, alcohol consumption, obesity, and some medications, can cause heartburn.

If heartburn pain is a frequent guest at your table, here are some things you can do to make your life more comfortable.

Eat less, more often. Small, frequent meals, say four to six light helpings a day, are healthier than three large ones. Avoid stuffing yourself and eating just before bedtime. Don't even lie down for four hours after eating.

Think bland. Fatty and spicy dishes will irritate your stomach lining and esophagus. Some of the worst offenders are tomato products, onions, and peppers. Acidic foods, like citrus juices, can also cause irritation.

Watch what you drink. Cut down on coffee, tea, alcoholic beverages, and whole milk. These tend to irritate your stomach lining.

Chew it to cool it. The more you chew, the more acid-neutralizing saliva you produce. Take small bites and chew your food slowly and thoroughly. After eating, chew a piece of sugarless gum. Sucking on sugarless hard candy during the day may also help, but avoid peppermint-flavored candy.

Timing is everything. Drink liquids about an hour before or after meals to keep your stomach from bloating. Don't mix foods and liquids.

Improve your posture. Sit up straight when you're eating — never stand or lie down. And don't bend over immediately after eating. This forces food and digestive acids back up into your esophagus.

Avoid tight clothes. Don't wear clothes and belts that fit tightly around your stomach. Choose clothes that fit loosely at your waistline.

Slim down. If you are overweight, losing those extra pounds may help relieve your symptoms. The extra weight squeezes your belly and forces the acidic digestive juices back up into your esophagus.

Do one thing at a time. Don't eat while working, playing, or driving.

Give up smoking. And if you're already trying to quit, don't wear your nicotine patch to bed. The nicotine it releases can cause heartburn.

Get support while you sleep. Use 4- to 6-inch wooden blocks or bricks to raise the head of your bed. Or, put a foam wedge beneath your upper body. This keeps digestive juices flowing down instead of up as you sleep. Extra pillows usually won't do the trick. They merely force a bend at your waist.

Turn to the left. A recent study found that sleeping on your left side may reduce your chances of getting heartburn. People in the study who slept on their backs had more episodes of heartburn than others. However, the stomach acid took longer to clear out of the esophagus in those who slept on their right sides — allowing more time for the acid to damage the esophagus.

Down the hatch. Drink plenty of water with your medications, and don't lie down after swallowing a pill. This helps the pills go down and stay down. Drinking water throughout the day will also help keep the digestive acids washed out of your esophagus.

Take it easy. Avoid straining and heavy lifting. This causes your abdominal muscles to contract and squeeze the contents of your stomach into your esophagus.

Know your medications. Talk to your doctor if you are taking any heart or blood pressure medicines. These can affect the sphincter between your esophagus and stomach, allowing acid to back up into your esophagus.

If your heartburn becomes severe and is accompanied by nausea, sweating, weakness, fainting, or breathlessness, or pain that extends from your chest to your arm or jaw, you may have something much worse than a pepperoni pizza that didn't sit well. These are symptoms of a heart attack. Call for emergency help.

How to use antacids wisely

When you're feeling the burn of heartburn, antacids may cool the fire in your chest, but they can have unpleasant side effects.

Always check the label before buying an antacid. Seltzer-type products contain a lot of salt and shouldn't be taken by people who are on low-sodium diets. Antacids high in calcium should be avoided by people with kidney problems. Calcium antacids can also cause a rebound effect, resulting in even greater acid production.

Be especially careful with magnesium-containing antacids. Don't take more than the recommended daily dose, and don't use them for more than a week without your doctor's approval. Otherwise, you could build up deadly levels of magnesium in your body. The signs of this dangerous side effect are low blood pressure, muscle weakness, lightheadedness, confusion, heart rhythm disturbances, nausea, and vomiting. The elderly are especially vulnerable.

Besides checking your antacid for these ingredients, consider switching from the liquid type to the tablet form. Research has found that tablets actually provide greater and longer-lasting relief than liquids.

A study of 65 heartburn sufferers revealed that Tums E-X tablets and Mylanta Double Strength tablets controlled heartburn better than the liquid Mylanta II and Extra Strength Maalox.

The tablets did a better job of lowering acid levels and reducing the number of times stomach juices flowed back into the esophagus. In fact, two hours after taking the medicine, only people who had used the liquid antacids were still having heartburn.

The tablets mix with your saliva to form a gummy substance that sticks to your esophagus better and longer than the liquid medicine. Plus, the act of chewing the tablets may bring out the natural antacids in your saliva.

Heatstroke

Surviving temperature extremes

Bad weather can be more than an inconvenience, especially if you're elderly. Weather can be dangerous, and it doesn't take a tornado or a hurricane to be deadly. Extreme heat and extreme cold can affect your heart, and they can sometimes be fatal.

Heat-related illnesses kill almost 400 people every year in the United States, according to the Centers for Disease Control (CDC). Infants and people over 65 are at greatest risk.

When it's hot, your body sweats to cool off. This causes you to lose fluid, which decreases your blood volume. Your heart has to work harder to pump the reduced amount of blood throughout your body. Then, if you exercise outdoors in hot weather, you're doubling the strain on your heart.

You should know the symptoms of heat exhaustion and heatstroke and take steps immediately to cool down.

Symptoms of heat exhaustion include heavy sweating; cold, clammy skin; dizziness; rapid heartbeat; headache; and nausea. If heat exhaustion progresses to heatstroke, your body, including your heart and brain, will begin to shut down. A high fever, slow pulse, low blood pressure, gray skin, and confusion are some of the symptoms of heatstroke.

During a heat wave, limit outdoor activities and stay in an air-conditioned building, especially if you're elderly or have a heart condition. Drink lots of nonalcoholic fluids and take cool baths.

Weather that is too cold can also be dangerous because it can cause hypothermia, a severely reduced body temperature. This happens because your body can't produce enough energy to keep your internal temperature warm enough. Symptoms of this potentially fatal condition include confusion, sleepiness, and lack of coordination. Heart failure is the most common cause of death in cases of hypothermia.

Protect yourself from hypothermia in cold weather by wearing layers of clothing, a hat, and gloves or mittens. A hat is especially important. Also, don't drink alcohol before going out into the cold. You may think it's warming you up, but it's actually drawing warmth from your internal organs to your skin, making you more vulnerable to hypothermia.

● ●
The sweet smell of sweat

You may hate to do it, but sweating is good for you. Your body's 3 million sweat glands perform an important task — helping to regulate your body temperature.

Step outside on a hot day, and your body immediately begins to cool itself. Tiny blood vessels in your skin dilate, expanding their surface area to dissipate heat. Your sweat glands pull water from your blood and send it to your skin, bathing you in cooling sweat.

According to scientists, sweat that is the result of heat is odorless — it's emotional sweating that's stinky.

No matter what's making you sweat, if you want to smell good, your diet can help. Certain vegetables, like parsley, contain chlorophyll, a natural deodorant that helps prevent body odor. And other foods, like garlic, onions, and some cheeses, can make your body — and your breath — smell badly.

● ●

Hemorrhoids

Relief for hemorrhoids

Hemorrhoids are a real pain. These swollen veins can occur inside the rectum or bulge outside the anus. Both kinds can become itchy and painful, and they can also bleed.

There's no reason to live with the pain. Give these natural remedies a try, but if your condition worsens or doesn't improve within seven days, or if bleeding occurs, see your doctor.

Fight back with fiber. The number one way to prevent and treat hemorrhoids is to add fiber to your diet. Fiber will help you avoid constipation, soften your stool, and relieve the pressure on your hemorrhoids.

Try to get about 25 to 30 grams of fiber each day. Good sources are bran, whole grain foods, potatoes, beans, and fresh fruits. To really get things moving, eat more cabbage, corn, parsnips, brussels sprouts, cauliflower, peas, asparagus, carrots, and kale.

Take it "sitzing" down. If your hemorrhoids are inflamed, soaking in a few inches of warm water with your knees raised will really ease your pain. Try three 15-minute soaks a day to soothe your uncomfortable symptoms. Don't make the water too hot, and don't add anything like bubble bath or Epsom salts — these can irritate swollen veins. You can relax in your tub or find Sitz Baths at your local pharmacy for a reasonable price.

Practice proper bathroom etiquette. Straining during a bowel movement is one of the major causes of hemorrhoids. To prevent this, take a footstool into the bathroom and prop up your feet. If you don't have a stool, anything that raises your feet at least a few inches will help.

Before having a bowel movement, try gently lubricating the area, inside and out, with a water-based lubricant, like K-Y Jelly (not petroleum jelly), to ease irritation.

And although you shouldn't rush the process, don't sit too long either. Enjoying your favorite magazine for more than a few minutes increases the pressure on the veins in your rectum. The longer you sit, the more your veins swell.

Last, but not least, clean well. If the area is particularly sensitive after a bowel movement, wipe with a soft, moist tissue or baby wipes instead of regular toilet tissue.

Flush it out. Six to eight glasses of liquid each day will flush out your digestive system. Stay away from alcohol because it draws water from your body and causes constipation.

Stay active. Hemorrhoids should not restrict your normal exercise routine. In fact, it's more important than ever for you to exercise every day — for two reasons. First of all, moving around instead of sitting takes pressure off the veins in your rectum. And secondly, exercise helps prevent constipation, one of the main causes of hemorrhoids. Just avoid heavy lifting and any activity that causes you to strain.

Slim down. Being overweight is often a consequence of an inactive lifestyle and poor diet. Changing these two aspects of your life will improve your health, including the condition of your hemorrhoids.

Cool the heat. If your hemorrhoids are painfully swollen, take this as an excuse to rest. Stay in bed for a few hours with an ice pack on your anal area.

Reach for over-the-counter help. There are several products you can buy for different kinds of hemorrhoid relief. Bulk stool softeners are helpful, but stay away from laxatives. Diarrhea is just as bad for hemorrhoids as constipation. If you choose a commercial product, these are some helpful ingredients:

- Hydrocortisone — relieves inflammation and itching.

- Anesthetics (benzocaine, pramoxine) — can numb the pain.

- Vasoconstrictors (ephedrine, phenylephrine) — reduce swelling and relieve itching.

- Astringents (witch hazel, zinc oxide) — help shrink blood vessels.

- Counterirritants (camphor) — soothe and comfort the area.

- Aloe vera gel — reduces irritation.

Particular brands may list other ingredients, such as wound-healing agents and antiseptics, but not all of these have been proven useful.

Hiccups

15 hiccup remedies that really work

Man can walk on the moon and create computers the size of a fingernail, but curing hiccups still remains a mystery. Although doctors have tried everything from drugs to hypnosis, these old-fashioned home remedies really work.

Change the pressure in your sinuses. By plugging up your ear canal, you are increasing the pressure inside your sinuses. This could force the muscle spasm that caused the hiccup to relax.

- plug up one ear with your finger
- plug both ears and drink a glass of water

Master some massage therapy. Many experts believe the upper part of your spinal column, in the back of your neck, controls hiccups. Several of these remedies apply pressure to nerve centers that may be connected to this control site.

- pull gently on your tongue
- with a spoon, lift the uvula (the small tissue hanging down at the back of your throat)
- pinch your upper lip, just below your right nostril
- apply gentle pressure to your closed eyelids

Stimulate your throat. The nerves at the back of your throat may trigger the muscle spasm causing your hiccups. By distracting those nerves with something else, you may be able to stop the hiccups.

- sip ice water

- gargle

- swallow some sugar

- bite on a lemon

Check your breathing. The idea is to interrupt the hiccup cycle by stopping the flow of oxygen for a short time.

- draw your knees to your chest and wrap your arms around them and squeeze

- hold your breath

- sneeze

- cough

- breathe into a paper bag

High blood pressure

5 drug-free ways to lower blood pressure

High blood pressure shouldn't be taken lightly. It can affect almost every organ in your body and increases your risk of heart attack, stroke, kidney damage, aneurysms, vision problems, and memory loss. Have your blood pressure checked regularly, and if your doctor prescribes medication, follow his instructions.

Here are some other things you can do to help keep your blood pressure under control.

Drop a little weight. The number one thing you can do to lower your blood pressure is to lose weight. Even losing just a few pounds can substantially reduce your risk of developing high blood pressure. One recent study found that women who had a BMI of 31 or more (*See BMI chart in the Weight gain chapter.*) were more than six times as likely to develop high blood pressure as women with BMIs less than 20. Even women with a BMI of 20 to 20.9 had a significantly higher risk. In fact, a one point increase in BMI was associated with a 12-percent increase in risk for high blood pressure.

In the study, women who lost between two and four and a half pounds lowered their risk by 15 percent, and women who lost more than four and a half pounds lowered their risk by 26 percent.

Take a daily walk. Getting regular exercise can help you lose weight. It can also lower your blood pressure and keep your arteries flexible. As you age, your blood vessels become less flexible. When your muscles need more oxygen and nutrients, your arteries can't dilate to allow more blood to flow through. Your heart has to work harder, which increases your heart rate and blood pressure. By exercising regularly, you are actually keeping your arteries in shape, not just your muscles.

Getting regular exercise doesn't have to be difficult. One study in Japan found that men who walked to work had a reduced risk of developing high blood pressure. Those who walked longer had even less risk. If you don't live where you can walk to work, at least try parking farther away and walking some of the distance. And if you don't work, make time each day for a 20-minute walk.

Cool your temper. When you get really angry, can you feel your blood pressure shooting skyward? Studies show that if you learn to control anger and hostility, you can help control your blood pressure. In a recent study, one group of people attended eight weekly group therapy sessions designed to teach them how to express anger in an appropriate manner. A second "control" group was not involved in any anger-management program. At the end of the study, the average diastolic blood pressure (bottom number) in the therapy group had been reduced from 90.3 to 85.2. Two months later, the average reading had dropped even more — to 81.8. The average diastolic blood pressure of the people in the control group was higher at the end of the study — 94.4, up from 88.9. After two months, the control group's average had risen to 95.

Meditate. One time-tested way of managing stress and anger is meditation. Scientific studies have shown that meditation can also lower blood pressure.

One recent study tested 32 healthy adults, 18 of whom had been practicing meditation for years. When the people were instructed to rest with their eyes open, the average systolic blood pressure (top number) of the meditators fell by about two and a half points, compared with a half-point rise in the other group. Then, the meditation group meditated with eyes closed for 20 minutes, while the other group was told to close their eyes and relax as completely as possible. The meditation group experienced an average drop in systolic pressure of three points compared with an average two point rise in the nonmeditating group.

Get a pet. Your canine companion or feline friend may help keep your blood pressure under control. A recent study looked at 48 male and female stockbrokers who were taking medication for high blood pressure. When placed under stress, the blood pressure of those with a pet rose, but only by about half as much as those without a pet.

● ●
Benefits of exercise last for hours

Exercise is one of the best ways to lose weight and lower your blood pressure. Now a new study reveals even more good news.

The study found that blood pressure was lower even hours after exercising. After three 15-minute sessions on a treadmill, reductions in systolic blood pressure remained for 16 hours, and reductions in diastolic blood pressure remained for 12 hours.

Average blood pressure readings were lower overall for the 24-hour period following exercise than on days when the men didn't exercise.

This means your heart doesn't have to work quite as hard for hours after you exercise. So give your heart a break and take a hike, go for a walk, ride a bike, fly a kite — just move it.

● ●

DASH high blood pressure in 2 weeks

Be careful what you put on your plate. Your eating habits can contribute to the development of high blood pressure. Luckily, researchers have found an eating plan that can reduce high blood pressure in as little as two weeks.

A scientific study called "DASH" (Dietary Approaches to Stop Hypertension) found that high blood pressure was reduced when people ate less saturated fat, total fat, and cholesterol and more fruits, vegetables, and low-fat dairy foods.

Researchers compared three eating plans:

- A typical American diet

- A diet similar to the first but containing more fruits and vegetables

- The DASH diet, which was low in saturated fat, total fat, and cholesterol and rich in fruits, vegetables, and low-fat dairy foods

People on the DASH diet reduced their systolic blood pressure an average of six points and their diastolic blood pressure an average of three points. In the people who had high blood pressure, systolic dropped by 11 points and diastolic dropped by six points. This reduction occurred within just two weeks of starting the diet.

The really good news is that the DASH diet isn't hard to follow. The National Heart, Lung, and Blood Institute (NHLBI) offers these tips for beginning the DASH plan.

- Change gradually. If you now eat one or two vegetables a day, add a serving at lunch and another at dinner.

- If you don't eat fruit now or have only juice at breakfast, add a serving to your meals or have it as a snack.

- Use only half the butter, margarine, or salad dressing you do now.

- Try low-fat or fat-free condiments, such as mayonnaise and salad dressings.

- Gradually increase dairy products to three servings per day. For example, drink milk with lunch or dinner instead of soda, alcohol, or sugar-sweetened tea. Choose low-fat (1 percent) or fat-free (skim) dairy products to reduce total fat intake.

- Limit meat, poultry, and fish to two 3-ounce servings a day or less. A 3-ounce serving is about the size of a deck of cards.

- If you now eat large portions of meat, cut them back gradually — by a half or a third at each meal. Treat meat as one part of the whole meal, instead of the focus.

- Include two or more vegetarian meals each week.

- Increase servings of vegetables, rice, pasta, and dry beans in your meals.

- Try casseroles, pasta, and stir-fry dishes with less meat and more vegetables, grains, and dry beans.

- Use fruits or low-fat foods as desserts and snacks. Buy fruits canned in their own juice. Fresh fruits require little or no preparation. Dried fruits are easy to carry with you.

- Try these snack ideas — unsalted pretzels or nuts mixed with raisins, graham crackers, low-fat and fat-free yogurt and frozen yogurt, plain popcorn with no salt or butter added, and raw vegetables.

Because the DASH diet has more daily servings of fruits, vegetables, and grains than most people are used to, the increase in fiber could cause bloating and diarrhea. To avoid this, increase your servings of fruits, vegetables, and grains gradually.

Although you may see results in just two weeks, the DASH diet is really an eating plan for life. You must change your eating habits permanently if you want lower blood pressure.

For more information about the DASH diet, write to: NHLBI Information Center, PO Box 30105, Bethesda, MD 20824-0105. If you have Internet access, you can also visit this Web site: <http://dash.bwh.harvard.edu>.

Vitamin C joins the battle

Lower your blood pressure and put the spring back in your arteries with vitamin C — at least that's what some researchers are saying.

In a recent study, people with high blood pressure who took a 500-milligram (mg) supplement of vitamin C each day for a month reduced their blood pressure by almost 10 percent. People in the study who took a placebo also reduced their blood pressure, but only by about 3 percent.

Another study found that after people took vitamin C, their arteries became significantly less stiff, and their platelets were less sticky, reducing the risk of blood clots. The people taking a placebo experienced no change.

Vitamin C is a potent antioxidant, and researchers believe it protects your body's supply of nitric oxide, which helps blood vessels relax.

While more research is needed to confirm these findings, most people would benefit by eating foods rich in vitamin C. Citrus fruits, strawberries, sweet red peppers, and green peppers are excellent sources.

• •

Turn back the clock

If you need an incentive to keep your blood pressure under control, a recent study of elderly men might provide it.

The study found that certain risk factors speed up your brain's aging — and high blood pressure and smoking topped the list.

As you age, nerve tissue in your brain becomes damaged and your brain shrinks. This accounts for some of the loss of mental abilities in older people.

And yet, if you take care of your health, especially by keeping your blood pressure under control, you can limit the amount of damage and shrinkage. Researchers estimate that high blood pressure and other risk factors accounted for about 15 percent of the abnormal tissue in brain structure in the study participants.

• •

Crunchy way to help lower your blood pressure

Crunching celery might do more for you than satisfy your appetite. Celery, an old Oriental remedy for mild hypertension, apparently is still effective.

Scientists discovered that celery contains a chemical that opens the blood vessels, which in turn lowers your blood pressure. Researchers caution against using the celery cure alone. Celery contains sodium and other chemicals, which at high doses can be harmful to your body. Check with your doctor about including more celery in your diet.

Don't let drug side effects side line you

Some people need medication to lower their blood pressure and prevent complications. If you're one of them, you should know the type of drug you are taking and what side effects you might experience. Ask your doctor to provide you with complete information on the medicine he prescribes. These are some of the more common types of medicine for high blood pressure.

ACE inhibitors. ACE stands for angiotensin converting enzyme. ACE inhibitors work by blocking a chemical called angiotensin in your body that causes blood vessels to tighten. As a result, ACE inhibitors relax your blood vessels. This lowers your blood pressure and increases the supply of blood and oxygen to your heart. A recent study found that ACE inhibitors also improved people's chances of surviving after a heart attack.

Side effects include fatigue, headache, cough, and nausea. An allergic reaction to ACE inhibitors, or any drug, can be very serious. If you experience any swelling, especially your tongue or throat, seek medical help immediately.

Beta blockers. These drugs lower blood pressure by blocking certain actions of your sympathetic nervous system. They expand blood vessel walls and slow down the contractions of your heart.

Possible side effects include fatigue, dizziness, headache, breathing difficulty, nausea, diarrhea, asthma, and insomnia.

Calcium channel blockers. These drugs work by affecting the movement of calcium into the cells of your heart and blood vessels. They relax your blood vessels and increase the blood and oxygen supply to your heart.

Controversy surrounds the use of calcium channel blockers, mostly the short-acting ones. A recent study found that post-menopausal women who took calcium channel blockers were twice as likely to develop breast cancer as other women. Other studies have found an increase in deaths and heart attacks among people taking short-acting nifedipine, a calcium channel blocker.

The National Heart, Lung, and Blood Institute recommends to doctors that "short-acting nifedipine should be used with great caution (if at all), especially at higher doses in the treatment of hypertension (high blood pressure), angina, and MI (myocardial infarction)." The American Heart Association cautions people who are already taking this drug not to suddenly stop taking it without consulting their doctors.

Diuretics. These work on your kidneys to increase urination and get rid of excess fluid. They are probably the most commonly recommended high blood pressure medication — and the most inexpensive.

One problem with diuretics is that you may be flushing out too many minerals with your urine, including potassium, which is important for your heart's health. If you are taking a diuretic, your doctor may recommend potassium supplements, or he can prescribe a potassium-sparing diuretic.

Loop diuretics are another type of diuretic. They are so-named because they work in a part of the kidney called the Loop of Henle. This makes them more effective.

Whatever medication your doctor prescribes, make sure you follow his instructions carefully.

● ●
'Sawing logs' risk factor for disease

If your spouse wears earplugs to bed, your health could be in danger. Snoring and sleep apnea may increase your risk of heart disease, stroke, and high blood pressure.

One study found that women who snore regularly were twice as likely to die from heart attacks or strokes. Women who snore occasionally were almost 50 percent more likely to have a heart attack or stroke and 61 percent more likely to die from them.

Another study on men and women found that people with sleep apnea (a disorder in which you stop breathing momentarily in your sleep, then snort and gasp for air) were significantly more likely to have high blood pressure. Each episode of sleep apnea per hour of sleep added about 1 percent to the risk of having high blood pressure.

Sleep apnea can be treated. If you have this condition, see your doctor. And while you may not be able to stop your snoring, be aware that you are at higher risk for heart disease. This means you should do everything you can to eliminate other risk factors.

● ●

The latest word on the salt controversy

If you follow the advice of most government health organizations, you're probably not shaking much salt onto your foods. The National Heart, Lung, and Blood Institute (NHLBI) recommends no more than 2,400 milligrams (mg) of sodium a day. Yet, some researchers disagree with the government recommendations. At the American Association for the Advancement of Science's annual conference, scientists questioned the findings of Intersalt, one of the landmark studies those recommendations are based on.

Intersalt, a huge international study done in 1988, found a link between sodium intake and high blood pressure. Usually, the more salt you eat, the more you excrete in your urine. Intersalt found that people with a high-sodium content in their urine were more likely to have high blood pressure. The association was stronger for older people.

Some scientists question the way the information from Intersalt was interpreted and say new studies provide more reliable information.

More recent studies have found that only about 20 to 30 percent of the people have blood pressure that fluctuates with salt intake — and not everyone responds to salt with an increase in blood pressure. The people who do are called salt-sensitive. These are the people who really need to watch their salt intake.

How do you know if you're salt-sensitive? Right now, the only way to be sure is to monitor your blood pressure and salt intake carefully over a period of time to see if eating salt raises your blood pressure. This can be a very time-consuming process, but if you'd like to know if you're salt-sensitive, you can try this three-step test.

1. Record your blood pressure and salt intake under normal circumstances.

2. Restrict salt to 2,000 mg a day and record your blood pressure.

3. Increase salt by 1,000 mg a day to determine when more salt causes your blood pressure to rise.

One study of 27 men found that some of the men with normal blood pressure were "salt-resistant," which means their blood pressure didn't automatically fall when they reduced their salt intake. In fact, blood pressure increased by as much as five points in some men who reduced their salt intakes.

Many of the men in the study had high levels of insulin, suggesting that the body may adapt to a low-salt diet by producing more insulin. Studies have shown that insulin can contribute to hardening of the arteries by encouraging the body to produce excess cholesterol. Insulin also encourages your kidneys to retain salt.

The scientists who disagree with the government's recommendations on salt intake aren't saying that people should eat more salt. Most people probably get more than they need in their everyday diets. The scientists believe that a blanket recommendation to reduce salt intake isn't the best way to reduce blood pressure. They say weight loss is still the best and most well-established method of lowering blood pressure.

High cholesterol

Ancient Chinese remedy lowers cholesterol

The Chinese have had an effective cholesterol-lowering substance in their diet for centuries. Known as red yeast rice, it's used as a flavoring in dishes like Peking duck.

Red yeast rice is made by fermenting a certain type of yeast on a bed of rice. Records indicate the Ancient Chinese believed this yeast could improve heart health. Modern researchers in China tested the effectiveness of this ancient remedy to confirm its cholesterol-lowering powers.

In one study, researchers gave 600 milligrams (mg) of red yeast rice twice a day or 1,200 mg of a Chinese herb reputed to have cholesterol-lowering properties to people with high cholesterol. After eight weeks of treatment, the people taking the red yeast rice reduced their total cholesterol an average of 22 percent. The people taking the herb had an average reduction of only 7 percent.

In the United States, research also supports the effectiveness of red yeast rice. Pharmanex, a company that manufactures Cholestin, the first red yeast rice supplement marketed in the United States, helped fund a double-blind study of Cholestin's effectiveness at the University of California at Los Angeles. Researchers gave participants 2.4 grams of Cholestin daily or a placebo. After eight weeks, the people taking the Cholestin experienced an 18-percent decrease in their cholesterol levels, and the people taking the placebo experienced no change.

Other brands of red yeast rice supplements are now available in health food stores, drugstores, through mail order, and on the Internet.

If you decide to try a red yeast rice supplement, don't mix it with your prescription cholesterol-lowering drug. And don't stop taking your prescribed medication without consulting your doctor. Talk with him and tell him you want to try red yeast rice. If he agrees it's worth a try, ask to have your cholesterol levels checked to see if the supplement is as effective for you as your prescription.

Although no serious side effects have been documented with the use of red yeast rice, because it is similar to statin drugs, it may cause some of the same side effects. According to manufacturer's warning, you shouldn't take red yeast rice if you:

- are at risk for liver disease, have active liver disease, or any history of liver disease

- consume more than two drinks of alcohol a day

- have a serious infection

- have undergone an organ transplant

- have a serious disease or physical disorder or have recently undergone major surgery

If you prefer the totally natural form, look for red yeast rice at specialty stores that carry Chinese foods. The natural product isn't standardized, so you won't know exactly how much you're getting. Don't substitute it for your prescription cholesterol-lowering drug. However, if you add it to your regular diet, and it seems to affect your cholesterol levels favorably, you may be able to cut back on your medication, with your doctor's guidance and approval.

• •
Cholesterol vaccine on the horizon

If you have a hard time keeping your cholesterol under control, help is on the way.

A cholesterol vaccine designed to prevent your body from converting good HDL cholesterol to bad LDL cholesterol may be available soon. The vaccine attaches a toxin to a protein necessary for the conversion of HDL to LDL.

Studies done on animals found that those given the vaccine had 35 percent higher HDL cholesterol levels. Lesions in arteries were also reduced by about 40 percent. Results from human studies aren't available yet.

Researchers say the vaccine would be given two or three times a year, which would be easier for most people than taking pills every day.

Check with your doctor to see when this vaccine will be available.

• •

Choose foods that cut cholesterol

If your doctor says your cholesterol is too high, you have lots of company. About half the people in the United States have cholesterol levels at least slightly above the desirable level of 200. And, according to a recent study, lowering that figure by just 10 percent would result in a 20-percent decrease in heart attack deaths. That's a great reason to get your cholesterol under control.

A good way to start is by maintaining a healthy weight and eating less saturated fat — not always easy tasks. Luckily, adding these things to your diet can help clobber cholesterol, too.

Orange juice. A glass of orange juice at each meal can increase your good HDL cholesterol. A recent study found that people who drank three glasses of orange juice a day raised their HDL levels by 21 percent and lowered the ratio of bad LDL to good HDL cholesterol by 16 percent. Orange juice increased folate levels, too. Folate, also called folic acid, is known to fight homocysteine, a heart disease risk factor.

Garlic. If you like to use this pungent bulb in your favorite dishes, you may be doing your arteries a favor.

Dozens of studies have found that garlic prevents the build up of fat and cholesterol in your arteries, reduces triglycerides, and increases HDL cholesterol. In one of those studies, eating a fresh clove of garlic every day for 16 weeks reduced cholesterol by an amazing 20 percent.

Fiber. Fiber helps lower LDL cholesterol and may even raise HDL cholesterol. Fiber also fills you up, leaving less room for meat and dairy products high in cholesterol and fat. Bran, oats, barley, wild rice, hominy, and flaxseed are good sources of fiber. Legumes, like split peas, black-eyed peas, lentils, kidney beans, and soybeans, are another inexpensive way to add fiber to your meals. And don't forget fruits and vegetables. They make great snacks and are loaded with fiber.

If you get the bulk of your fiber from bread, rye might be a better choice for lowering cholesterol than wheat. One study found that men with high cholesterol levels who ate rye bread lowered total cholesterol by 8 percent. Eating wheat bread didn't make any measurable difference in their cholesterol levels.

Yogurt. Some bacteria can be good for you. Yogurt fermented by certain kinds of bacteria may reduce your cholesterol levels. Experts have debated yogurt's ability to lower cholesterol for years. Researchers analyzed the results of several studies and came to the conclusion that several fermented dairy products were effective in lowering cholesterol, including yogurt and milk products that contain bifidus or acidophilus. Other cholesterol-lowering foods include fermented vegetables and kefir, a fermented dairy product.

Lean meat. For years, doctors have been telling people with high cholesterol to avoid red meat. However, during a recent study, researchers put people with high cholesterol on an eating plan that included either lean red meat, like beef, veal, or pork, or white meat, like fish or chicken. At the end of the study, changes in cholesterol levels between the two groups were almost the same.

If you do include red meat in your diet, choose lean cuts, trim off any excess fat, and use low-fat cooking methods, like broiling, roasting, or grilling. After cooking ground beef, blot it with paper towels and rinse it in hot water to remove as much fat as possible.

●●●●●●●●●●●●●●●●●●●●●●●●●●●●●

Butter vs. margarine

Butter is high in cholesterol and saturated fat. Margarine is cholesterol-free and is usually made from unsaturated liquid vegetable oil — but it's not perfect.

When vegetable oils are hardened during a process called hydrogenation, trans fatty acids are formed. These trans fatty acids have the same effect in the body as saturated fat. They raise cholesterol levels.

To help you make a choice, consider the latest American Heart Association recommendations:

• Choose a margarine with no more than 2 grams of saturated fat per tablespoon.

• Look for a margarine with liquid vegetable oil listed as the first ingredient.

• Buy soft margarine instead of stick.

The new margarine substitutes that help lower cholesterol may be an even better choice. The low-fat spreads are made from vegetable oil with added sterol esters. Sterol esters are made from plant oils, and because they are structurally similar to cholesterol, they interfere with the body's absorption of cholesterol.

These spreads seem to lower bad LDL cholesterol without lowering good HDL cholesterol. One kind, called Benecol, is made from sitostanol ester, a by-product of the wood processing industry. Studies show this margarine resulted in a 20-percent drop in LDL cholesterol by blocking absorption of some cholesterol into the bloodstream. Another kind, called Take Control, is made from plant sterols extracted from soybeans.

• •

E-Z way to protect your arteries

Can something as simple as taking a daily vitamin protect your heart from disease? Several studies indicate that vitamin E helps prevent bad LDL cholesterol from becoming oxidized, which contributes to the buildup of artery-clogging plaque.

Vitamin E may be particularly effective in protecting fats from becoming oxidized because it is a fat-soluble vitamin. Numerous studies have found that vitamin E can help protect your heart and blood vessels from free radical damage, which helps prevent heart disease.

One study from the Harvard School of Public Health found that men who had taken at least 100 international units (IU) of vitamin E a day for at least two years had 37 percent fewer heart attacks than men who didn't take vitamin E supplements. Another study found that women who took vitamin E supplements for more than two years had 41 percent fewer heart attacks.

Those studies were done on people who had no history of heart disease. The Cambridge Heart Antioxidant Study (CHAOS) was designed to find out if vitamin E could help people who already had heart disease.

Researchers gave the study participants 400 or 800 IU of vitamin E daily. After about 200 days of treatment, the participants' risk of having a nonfatal heart attack was reduced by 77 percent. Although the vitamin E didn't have an effect on death rates, the researchers pointed out that most deaths occurred early in the study, before the vitamin E would have had a chance to work.

On the other hand, a more recent study disputes the findings of these earlier studies. Researchers in Canada gave over 9,000 people either a supplement containing 400 IU of vitamin E or a placebo.

After four to six years, there was no significant difference in the number of people in each group who had a heart attack or stroke or died from these causes.

Researchers who conducted the study say that these results are a strong indication that vitamin E does not protect against heart disease. However, they note that everyone in the study had heart disease or diabetes and at least one other factor for a heart attack or stroke.

Despite the negative results of this study, the bulk of evidence still indicates that vitamin E can protect against heart disease.

If you decide to take vitamin E supplements, be aware that those made from natural sources are better absorbed by your body than synthetic ones. You can tell if a supplement contains natural or synthetic vitamin E by reading the label. Natural vitamin E is listed as "d" alpha-tocopherol and synthetic is listed as "dl" alpha-tocopherol.

Good food sources of vitamin E include wheat germ oil, olive oil, peanuts, almonds, and sunflower seeds.

● ●
Check your thyroid gland

Did you know high cholesterol could be caused by an underactive thyroid gland? If you didn't, you're not alone. A recent survey found that more than half the people surveyed who had been diagnosed with high cholesterol didn't know if they'd ever been tested for thyroid disease.

According to the American Association of Clinical Endocrinologists (AACE), diet is still the leading cause of high cholesterol — but thyroid disease comes in second.

● ●

Beware the dangers of low cholesterol

High cholesterol can be a warning that your heart is headed for trouble, but low cholesterol can be a warning sign of disease, too.

Research shows that people with low cholesterol are more likely to die from cancer and respiratory and digestive diseases — not diseases related to clogged arteries. One study found that people with low cholesterol also had low levels of antioxidants. Researchers believe low levels of antioxidants can put your body at greater risk of free radicals, which can damage cells and lead to disease.

Another study found that when elderly people have low cholesterol and low levels of albumin, a blood protein, their risk of dying goes up substantially. In the study of over 900 healthy people in their 70s, those with low albumin and low cholesterol levels were 3.6 times more likely to die within a 3-year period compared to those with higher levels.

Low cholesterol levels may also contribute to poor mental health. A recent study found that women with very low levels of cholesterol were more likely to suffer from depression and anxiety. More than a third of the women with low cholesterol scored high on tests designed to measure degrees of depression. Only about one-fifth of the women in the study with higher levels of cholesterol scored high on the depression scale.

These studies aren't suggesting that you should try to keep your cholesterol levels high. High cholesterol is a major risk factor for heart disease. If your doctor says your cholesterol levels are too low, talk with him about your diet and follow his advice.

Impotence

Start now to save your sex life

According to a survey conducted by the American Association of Retired Persons (AARP), 67 percent of men and 57 percent of women age 45 and older say a satisfying sexual relationship is important to their quality of life.

But your quality of life can take a sudden plunge if you have erectile dysfunction, more commonly known as impotence. Although almost every man has a problem once in a while, impotence is defined as a consistent inability to achieve and maintain an erection sufficient for sexual intercourse. If you develop impotence, take comfort in the fact that you are not alone. About 26 out of 1,000 men ages 40 to 69 develop impotence every year.

Because your erection depends on blood flow to your penis, anything that interferes with proper blood flow can cause impotence. People with diabetes, heart disease, or atherosclerosis (hardening of the arteries) are more likely to have the problem. Although your chances of having impotence rise as you get older, it is not an unavoidable consequence of aging.

Don't be embarrassed to talk with your doctor about sexual problems. There are many ways to treat impotence, but there are also ways to prevent it from happening in the first place. Since more than eight out of 10 cases of impotence can be traced to physical causes, taking care of yourself is one of the best ways to prevent it.

Watch the fat. High-fat foods can really foul up your sex life. Too much saturated fat and cholesterol in your diet can lead to high blood pressure and heart disease, which makes it harder for your blood vessels to get blood to where it needs to be during sex. In fact, a high total cholesterol count doubles a man's risk of becoming impotent. In one study, men whose cholesterol levels were higher than 240 were twice as likely to have impotence as those whose levels were below 180. It's also important to know that many of the medications prescribed for high blood pressure are known to cause impotence.

Keep your weight down. Excess weight could affect your sex life beyond just having unattractive "love handles." Too much weight can contribute to diabetes and high blood pressure, two major causes of impotence. About 40 percent of the men who have impotence are diabetics.

Stop smoking. If teenage boys knew what an effect smoking can have on their sex life as they get older, it might cut the rate of new smokers drastically. Research shows that just two cigarettes, smoked before intercourse, can significantly decrease blood flow to the penis. And long-term smokers are more likely to develop heart disease, which also contributes to impotence.

Limit alcohol. Drinking too much alcohol can cause even a young, healthy man to experience temporary impotence, and too much alcohol over several years can cause nerve and liver damage. This can lead to impotence that may be irreversible.

●●●●●●●●●●●●●●●●●●●●●●●●●●●●

Important warning sign of heart disease

Impotence may be frustrating, but if you pay attention, you could save your sex life — and your heart. Episodes of impotence could be an early warning of heart disease.

Researchers looked at test results of men who were impotent and found that 40 percent of them had significant blockages in their heart arteries. This is associated with an increased risk of heart attack, even though none of the men had symptoms of heart disease.

Because the arteries that supply the penis are small, they may be among the first to be affected by blockages that could later affect heart arteries.

The men in the study were lucky that their heart disease was discovered early. And many of them found that when they stopped smoking or lowered their cholesterol levels, their impotence went away.

So if you're normally sexually active and begin having problems, see your doctor.

• •

Sidestep bicycle-seat injuries

Bicycling is a great aerobic exercise, but you may be sitting on a hidden danger. Several studies show that bicycle seats can cause impotence; perineal (area between the anus and scrotum) numbness; and injuries to blood vessels, nerves, and other delicate tissue.

In a European study of long-distance male cyclists, 22 percent of the riders reported penile numbness and 13 percent reported impotence. In another study, 41 percent of weekend bike riders reported impotence. Surprisingly, 20 percent of riders of stationary exercise bikes suffered impotence, too.

Damage can occur when a narrow bike seat focuses your body's weight on the arteries and nerves that supply the pubic region. And for long-distance cyclists, that pressure may be exerted for long periods of time, increasing the risk of damage.

Problems with bikes aren't limited to men. At the American Urological Association in May 1999, studies were presented that suggested possible perineal injury from bicycling in both men and women.

Researchers at Boston University studied 282 female bikers ages 18 to 76. Of these women, 32 percent reported injuries from bicycle top tubes (the horizontal bar just below the seat) and 34 percent reported perineal numbness. Biking injuries can also cause urinary tract problems.

But don't put your bicycle up for sale just yet. Bicycling is still a healthy and enjoyable activity. Here are some steps you can take to lessen your risk of bicycle-seat injuries.

- Switch to a recumbent bike. You're seated lower on these bikes, and you lean back, with your back against a support. This means your weight is more evenly distributed.

- Get a new, ergonomic bike seat with a cut out area that completely takes the pressure off delicate nerves and arteries. These are available for about $50 in styles for men and women. Just visit your local bicycle shop.

- Get a wider bicycle seat, allowing your weight to be distributed more evenly.

- Rise out of your seat every 10 minutes and pedal for several minutes in a standing position.

- Change position frequently while riding.

- Adjust the handlebars and the height of the seat, making it horizontal or even pointing downward to take the pressure off. A knowledgeable employee in a bike shop can do this for you.

Irritable bowel syndrome

8 ways to control bowel trouble

It's one of the leading causes of employee absenteeism in the United States, and yet many people don't even know what it is — partly because most people are too embarrassed to discuss it.

Irritable bowel syndrome (IBS) is also known as "spastic colon" or "irritable colon," and is actually a set of chronic digestive symptoms. IBS symptoms include abdominal pain, frequent constipation and/or diarrhea, cramping, gas, and sometimes bloating, nausea, headache, and fatigue.

IBS affects more women than men, and symptoms usually begin in your 20s or 30s. It seldom begins after age 55. IBS isn't life-threatening, but it can make your life more difficult. Luckily, it usually can be controlled with a few diet and lifestyle changes.

Slow down. Everyone seems to be in a hurry these days, so mealtime may be a short affair. However, gulping down your food increases the chances that you might gulp air, too, so slow down and enjoy your food.

Steer clear of gas producers. Certain foods are more likely to cause you to have gas, which can aggravate your IBS. Limit your intake of beans, cabbage, onions, or any other food that has a tendency to make you react this way.

Can the carbonated drinks. Sodas and other carbonated drinks can also increase gas in your intestines, so limit your intake of those, too.

Manage your stress. By reducing stress in your life, you can give your digestive system a much-needed break. Your system is sensitive to stress, and many experts believe that stress and activities that tax your body in general are particularly harsh on your bowels. Try exercise or meditation to help manage your IBS symptoms.

Dodge the dairy. Although it may not affect you, lactose intolerance bothers about 40 percent of people with IBS. Look for ways to cut down on dairy products. More lactose-free products are being developed every day from such items as soy, rice, and even almonds.

Choose the right fiber. Fiber is essential to staying regular, but research suggests that bran and other grains may actually make IBS worse. Instead, try getting your fiber from gentler sources such as fruits and cooked vegetables. Researchers have found that these produce better results with far less chance of abdominal pain and bowel disturbance.

Psyllium, the dried seed husks of a certain type of plantain, is another natural way to help regulate yourself. It can be found in such over-the-counter products as Metamucil.

Keep a food diary. People with IBS may be more sensitive to certain foods. A good way to determine what foods cause flare-ups is to keep an IBS journal. When you experience symptoms, record what you have eaten recently as well as your activities and any stress you may be under. By keeping such a journal, you may see patterns forming and can prevent further outbreaks by avoiding their causes.

Try a little peppermint. For a natural way to relieve your bowel discomfort, try some peppermint oil. It may relax your intestinal muscles and soothe your cramps. If you take it as an enteric-coated capsule, it will dissolve in the intestines rather than the stomach, where it can irritate your stomach lining. Some IBS sufferers find relief by taking one to two 0.2 milliliter (ml) capsules three times a day, between meals.

Lung cancer

4 flavorful ways to beat lung cancer

If you never start smoking, you won't get lung cancer, right? Not necessarily. While smoking increases your risk of lung cancer dramatically, sometimes even nonsmokers get this deadly disease.

Previous research has shown that diet can greatly affect your risk of getting most cancers. But researchers found little evidence of a link between nutrition and lung cancer. Now they are discovering that certain foods and nutrients may indeed lower your risk for this deadliest of cancers.

Load up on onions, apples, and grapefruit. By now you probably know that flavonoids are substances found in plant-based foods that may help prevent certain diseases. A recent study found that two flavonoids, quercetin and naringin, might help prevent lung cancer. The main food sources of quercetin are onions and apples, and the main source of naringin is white grapefruit.

Make sure you get enough selenium. When researchers investigated selenium as a preventive for skin cancer, they discovered instead that this mineral might help prevent lung cancer.

The amount of selenium foods contain depends on the selenium content of the soil they were grown in. Foods that usually have enough include bran, broccoli, cabbage, celery, chicken, cucumbers, eggs, garlic, milk, mushrooms, and wheat germ.

Be careful about taking selenium supplements because too much selenium can be toxic if taken long-term. Never take more than 200 micrograms (mcg) of this mineral a day unless advised by a doctor.

Add some vitamin E. Vitamin E is a powerful antioxidant, and research finds that it may protect against many diseases, including lung cancer.

Information from one large cancer-prevention study suggests that high blood levels of vitamin E reduce lung cancer risk in smokers. The protective effect was strongest among people who had been smoking for less than 40 years, were under 60 years of age, and who took vitamin E supplements during the study.

Good food sources of vitamin E include wheat germ oil, sunflower seeds, almonds, mangoes, peanuts, and olive oil.

Try tofu or tempeh. Soy has been associated with a lower risk of hormone-related cancers, such as prostate and breast cancer. Preliminary studies indicate that a flavonoid found in soy, called genistein, may also protect against lung cancer.

Soybeans are legumes and are excellent sources of B vitamins, protein, and fiber. Tofu is probably the most well-known soy product. It usually comes in block form and has about the same weight and consistency as soft cheese. Tofu has almost no taste of its own and absorbs the flavor of whatever it is cooked with.

Other soy products include tempeh, which is a little firmer and more flavorful than tofu; miso, a salty seasoning paste often used in soups or ramen noodle products; soy flour; and soy milk.

Genistein content of soy products per half cup:

Soy flour	*50 mg*
Miso	*40 mg*
Tempeh	*40 mg*
Tofu	*40 mg*
Soybeans (cooked)	*35 mg*
Soy milk	*20 mg*

(New research claims soy may accelerate brain aging. For more information, see the *Mental impairment* chapter.)

• •

Cigars no safer than cigarettes

Cigar smoking has grown in popularity lately — it seems to be the "cool" thing to do. You may think that if you smoke cigars instead of cigarettes, you're not as likely to get lung cancer. After all, you probably don't even inhale the smoke.

Unfortunately, a new study pokes holes in that theory. It found that cigar smokers were five times as likely to die from lung cancer as nonsmokers. And those hardy souls who say they inhale the strong smoke are 11.3 times as likely to get the disease.

Cigar smokers also have a 45-percent higher risk of chronic obstructive lung disease, a 27-percent higher risk of heart disease, and about double the risk for cancers of the mouth, throat, and esophagus.

So stub out that stogie and save your lungs. It may just save your life.

• •

Smokers: Beware of these supplements

If you smoke, don't take beta carotene supplements. At least that's what researchers at the University of Texas Medical Branch are saying. Surprising news, considering experts have long considered antioxidants, like beta carotene, to be your body's first line of defense against cancer-causing free radicals. But a new study suggests beta carotene supplements may actually increase a smoker's risk of developing lung cancer.

In animal tests, beta carotene supplements increased the cancer-causing activity of cigarette smoke. When people were tested, heavy smokers taking beta carotene supplements had higher rates of lung cancer and lung cancer-related death.

This means when you smoke and take beta carotene supplements, the carcinogens in the cigarettes are even more active and dangerous, increasing your risk of cancer.

You may think this goes against everything you know about antioxidants and good health, but that's not so. The problem is people have forgotten that getting antioxidants from whole foods is different from taking supplements.

If you're thinking of loading up on antioxidant supplements to fight cancer or other diseases, think again — especially if you smoke. Instead, get your antioxidants from whole foods. The following is a list of foods containing antioxidants, like alpha-carotene; beta carotene; lutein; lycopene; and vitamins A, C, and E.

carrots	sweet potatoes	apricots	tomatoes
spinach	broccoli	mango	cantaloupe
watermelon	cress leaf	collard greens	parsley
pumpkin	meat	dairy citrus	nuts
peppers	wheat germ oil	sunflower seeds	

Menopause

Hormone replacement therapy — is it for you?

Some women may rejoice at the beginning of menopause because they don't have to deal with a menstrual period any more. Some women sail through menopause without a complaint. However, most women — about 75 percent — experience some unpleasant symptoms related to this condition.

These symptoms may include hot flashes, depression, sleep disturbances, inability to concentrate, and memory lapses. Your risk for bone fractures may increase because of a decrease in bone density, sex may become painful due to the thinning and drying of your vagina, and your skin may become drier and less elastic, resulting in more wrinkles. Your risk of heart disease also rises after menopause.

All these potential problems mean that menopause (for many women) centers around one decision — whether to begin hormone replacement therapy (HRT). Hormone replacement therapy isn't for everyone, but knowing the pros and cons will help you make an informed decision.

Heads off heart disease. The biggest benefit HRT offers may be a lower risk of heart disease. Before menopause, women are less likely to suffer heart disease than men, probably because of the protective effect of estrogen, but that risk increases dramatically after menopause. Heart disease is the number one killer of women over age 65.

Multiple studies have shown that women who use hormone replacement therapy have a 35- to 50-percent-lower risk of dying from heart disease. Scientists aren't sure exactly why, but studies show that HRT reduces low-density lipoprotein cholesterol and increases high-density lipoprotein cholesterol by 10 to 15 percent.

Hormone replacement therapy may be particularly beneficial to older women who smoke. A recent Australian study found that women smokers who had been on HRT for at least a year had much healthier arteries and lower cholesterol than the smokers not taking hormones.

Builds better bones. After menopause, women lose 1 to 8 percent of their skeleton every year. In fact, it's not unusual for a woman to lose one-third of her total bone mass within 10 years, leading to an increased risk of fractures, particularly hip fractures. Research finds that estrogen may reduce your fracture risk by more than 50 percent.

However, your lifestyle plays a big role in bone loss and in how much protection HRT may give you. Exercise protects against bone loss, while smoking and drinking alcohol increases fracture risk. A recent study found that HRT reduced the risk of hip fracture in smokers and former smokers, but not in women who had never smoked.

It also reduced fracture risk in women who drank alcohol and sedentary women, but not among nondrinkers and physically active women. In other words, you'll protect your bones if you exercise and don't drink excessively or smoke, but if you don't follow these good health practices, hormone replacement therapy may give you some protection.

Improves mind and mood. Sometimes it's difficult to tell if menopause is physically responsible for mind and mood problems like depression and forgetfulness because it occurs at a time of emotional changes for many women. Their reproductive years have come to an end, and children are growing up and leaving home. Nevertheless, studies suggest that estrogen may affect mood and mental abilities.

Recent studies have also shown that estrogen may improve depressed women's response to some antidepressant medications. One study at UCLA found that elderly depressed women on estrogen replacement therapy had almost a three times better chance of responding to Prozac.

Estrogen may also help you keep your mind sharp. A study at Stanford University found that women who took estrogen could remember names 39 percent better than women who didn't. Other studies suggest that estrogen use may even protect against Alzheimer's.

Maintains youthful skin. The elastic fibers that keep your skin tight change when they are deprived of estrogen. Taking estrogen may help strengthen these fibers and slow down the loss of collagen that occurs as you age. Research has shown that women with high levels of estrogen tend to appear much younger than their actual age, while those with low levels appear older.

In a recent study, researchers had men and women estimate the age of 100 women between the ages of 35 and 55. The women with high levels of estrogen were judged to looked younger, while women with low levels of the hormone were guessed to be older than they really were. The difference between real age and perceived age could be as high as eight years in either direction.

Preserves your smile. One reason for tooth loss as you age is that your bones, including your jawbone, may be giving way to osteoporosis. Estrogen may help keep your jawbone strong, and a recent study found that estrogen replacement therapy may lower gingival inflammation and the frequency of tooth loss.

Despite all these benefits, the long-term use of HRT remains controversial. The effects on women of taking supplemental estrogen for many years, even decades, is only beginning to be understood. Some research suggests an increased risk of breast cancer in women taking supplemental hormones. Research also finds that women on estrogen have an increased risk of endometrial cancer, but taking progestin with the estrogen prevents that increase in risk.

Talk to your doctor about the benefits and risks of hormone replacement so you can make a decision that's right for you.

• •
Over the hill and on the pill

Putting postmenopausal women on birth control pills may seem strange, but a recent study found that oral contraceptives boosted bone density, cut cholesterol, and lowered blood pressure better than regular hormone replacement therapy.

Oral contraceptives cost less than HRT, but because they contain higher levels of estrogen, can also cause more side effects. However, the pill could be a more effective, less expensive option for women with rapid bone loss. If your doctor recommends HRT, ask him about taking the pill instead.

• •

Making it through menopause the natural way

Prevention is usually the best treatment for any condition, and with menopause, prevention should begin long before you hit middle age. If you eat right, exercise, and don't smoke or drink excessively, you'll be in good shape, and your body will be better equipped to deal with the side effects of middle age. If you're already facing menopause, however, you can still take steps to minimize your symptoms and make the most of this time of your life.

Exercise. If you want menopause to be a breeze, make sure you exercise on a regular basis. Physical activity helps control weight and decreases your risk of heart disease and osteoporosis. Hot flashes are less common among physically active women than sedentary women. Exercise also enhances mental abilities, improves mood, and helps prevent insomnia.

The best exercise program for older women includes daily aerobic exercise like brisk walking, swimming, or bicycling; some type of resistance exercise, like weight training or even gardening, two to three times a week; and stretching exercises before and after the other activities. If this sounds like too much for you, remember to start slowly and don't give up. Even a little exercise is better than none.

Eat more soy. Plant estrogens — called phytoestrogens — are compounds found in some foods, particularly soy, that may be a natural way to boost your estrogen level after menopause.

Heart disease is one menopausal hazard that soy may help prevent. A recent study gave a soy-protein supplement, either once or twice daily, to perimenopausal women ages 45 to 55 years. The women who received the soy lowered their total and LDL cholesterol levels by about 5 to 7 percent compared to women who didn't receive soy.

Diastolic blood pressure was also significantly lower with the twice-daily soy diet. Women on the soy diet also reported that their hot flashes were less severe, although no less frequent.

Several studies have shown that soy can reduce the frequency and intensity of hot flashes but not as effectively as HRT. One study found that women using soy-protein supplements reported a 45-percent decrease in hot flashes. But the same study found that 30 percent of women given a placebo reported the same thing. Prescription estrogen, on the other hand, can reduce hot flashes 85 to 90 percent.

(New research claims soy may accelerate brain aging. For more information, see the Mental impairment chapter.)

Get help from the herb garden. Herbs can provide natural relief from some of the symptoms of menopause.

- **Depression.** Multiple studies have found that St. John's wort can effectively treat depression in some people, and it may help to relieve psychological symptoms like depression during menopause. One recent study gave women between 43 and 65 years of age one tablet of St. John's wort three times daily for 12 weeks. According to assessment tests, the women experienced improvement in psychological symptoms and in sexual well-being.

- **Insomnia.** Sleepless nights can be a common symptom of menopause, but some herbs may help. Valerian is an herb used extensively in Europe to treat insomnia. It may be particularly soothing as a warm bedtime tea. Just dissolve two teaspoons of dried valerian root in a cup of hot water for a night full of sweet dreams.

• •
Eat right to avoid fibroids

Here's a good reason to eat less red meat and more green vegetables — to reduce your risk of uterine fibroids.

Experts estimate that these benign tumors affect at least 20 to 30 percent of women in their reproductive years. Although fibroids aren't life-threatening, they can cause pelvic pain, anemia, and fertility problems.

A recent study found that women who ate the most red meat were 70 percent more likely to develop fibroids than women who ate the least amount of beef.

On the other hand, women who ate the most green vegetables had a 50 percent lower rate of fibroids, and women who ate the most fruit were 20 percent less likely to have them.

If you want to avoid this potentially painful condition, cut down on your intake of red meat, and beef up your intake of fruits and vegetables instead.

• •

Mental impairment

Soy linked to higher rates of senility

If you've started eating tofu burgers instead of hamburgers because you think soy is healthier — you may be in for a surprise. New research suggests that eating tofu may make your brain age faster, leading to serious problems with memory and learning in later years.

Even if you never eat tofu — a custard-like food made from pureed soybeans — you're still not in the clear. Soy or soybean oil can be found in everything from salad dressings, mayonnaise, and margarine to breakfast cereals and energy bars, making it the most widely used oil. It is estimated that soy protein is in 60 percent of all processed foods. And soy protein is added to the food of cattle and other livestock, so you may consume it indirectly just by eating your usual steak or hamburger.

Researchers in Hawaii concluded that soy may contribute to brain aging after examining the diets of more than 8,000 Japanese-American men for over 30 years. They found that those who ate two or more servings of tofu a week were much more likely to become senile or forgetful as they grew older compared with men who ate little or no tofu.

The more tofu the subjects ate, the more learning and memory problems they suffered in later life. Loss of mental function occurred in 4 percent of the men who ate the least amount of tofu compared with 19 percent of the men who ate the greatest amount of tofu.

These are shocking results for a food that has been touted for its health benefits and was recently given FDA approval to make health claims on package labels.

Dr. Lon White, lead researcher of the Hawaiian study, suggests the study's findings should make people think twice about the amount of soy they eat. "What we have here is a scary idea that may turn out to be dead wrong," he says. "Or it could turn out to be the first uncovering of an important health-negative effect of a food that we believe may have a lot of good going for it."

White's study included subjects ranging from 46 to 65 years old. The men were asked whether they ate certain foods associated with a traditional Japanese diet or an American diet. They were interviewed about their dietary habits again in the early 1970s and were tested for cognitive function — including attention, concentration, memory, language skills, and judgment — in the early 1990s when they were 71 to 93 years old. They were also given a brain scan at that time.

The results were disturbing. Out of 26 foods studied, only tofu was found to be significantly related to brain function. Men who had a high intake of tofu not only scored lower on tests of mental ability, but their brains were more likely to show signs of advanced age and shrinkage. Their test scores were typical of a person four years older.

Although the study was done on men, researchers also interviewed and tested 502 wives of the men in the study — and came up with similar findings.

The study has created a stir because it contradicts previous research that has found soy to be beneficial. Earlier studies have shown that soy may fight cancer and heart disease, prevent osteoporosis, and relieve menopause symptoms. Researchers credit estrogen-like molecules called isoflavones for soy's apparent disease-fighting properties. But those same substances could have negative effects on the body as well, White notes. He says people need to understand that isoflavones are complex chemicals that act like drugs and change the body's chemistry.

"The great things they [consumers] have been hearing about soy foods in recent years have little to do with nutrients — carbohydrates, proteins, fats, minerals, vitamins," he says. "All that hype is related to the idea that soy contains other kinds of molecules that act like medicines ... they alter the way our body chemistry works."

The isoflavones in soy are a type of phytoestrogen or plant estrogen, which mimics the estrogen produced naturally in your body. Brain cells have receptors that link up with estrogen to help maintain brain function, and White speculates that phytoestrogens may compete with the body's natural estrogens for these receptors.

Soy's isoflavones are also thought to interfere with enzymes and amino acids in the brain. One of soy's main isoflavones, genistein, has been shown to limit the enzyme tyrosine kinase in the hippocampus — the brain's memory center. By interfering with the activity of this enzyme, genistein blocks a process called "long-term potentiation" that is central to learning and memory.

Dr. Larrian Gillespie, author of *The Menopause Diet,* says eating too much soy could result in other problems as well. She has found that consuming 40 milligrams (mg) of isoflavones a day can slow down thyroid function, resulting in hypothyroidism. Most isoflavone supplements come in a 40-mg dose, and just 6 ounces of tofu or 2 cups of soy milk would supply the same amount.

Also, because isoflavones act like estrogen, some studies suggest that postmenopausal women who eat a lot of soy may increase their risk of breast cancer. And scientists have questioned the potential effects of soy on infants as well. One study found that infants who drank soy formula received six to 11 times as many phytoestrogens as the amount known to have hormonal effects in adults. Some think this could lead to early puberty, which is associated with a greater risk for breast cancer and ovarian cysts.

This leads to the question of whether soy's good aspects outweigh the negative ones.

"Whatever good effects come with the gift [soy], will also come at some cost," White says. "We do not know yet just what those costs are, just as we really don't know yet the full and honest extent of their health benefits. We're flying blind … and my data … are very, very disturbing."

The Hawaiian study was a long-term, well-designed, controlled study, but it was just one study. The results are strong enough to make everyone sit up and take notice, but more research needs to be done to confirm the results. If you eat soy, you may want to err on the side of caution. Be sure you know the amount of soy isoflavones you consume each day, and steer clear of soy supplements and soy-enriched foods (like some nutritional bars) until more research is done.

The chart on the next page will help you determine the isoflavone content of some common soy products.

How many soy isoflavones do you consume each day?

Food	Milligrams of isoflavones	*Serving size (approximate)
Bacon, meatless	1.9	2 strips (1/2 oz)
Granola bar (hard, plain)	.1	3.5 oz
Harvest Burger, (all vegetable protein patty)	8.2	1 patty
Infant formula, Prosobee® and Isomil® with iron, ready-to-feed	8	1 cup
Miso	43	1/2 cup
Peanuts, raw	0.3	1/2 cup
Soy breakfast links	(45 g)	1.7 2 links
Soy cheese, cheddar	7	3.5 ounce
Soy flour (textured)	148	1/2 cup
Soy hot dog (51 g)	3	2 hot dogs
Soy milk	20	1 cup
Soy powder (vanilla shake)	14 – 42 **	1 scoop
Soy protein nutritional bar	14 – 42 **	1 bar
Soy sauce, made from hydrolyzed vegetable protein	0.1	1/2 cup
Soy sauce, made from soy and wheat	1.6	1/2 cup
Soybean chips	54	1/2 cup
Soybeans (roasted)	128	1/2 cup
Tempeh	44	1/2 cup
Tofu (silken, firm)	28	1/2 cup
Tofu, yogurt	16	1/2 cup

USDA Commodity, beef patties with Vegetable Protein Product (VPP), frozen, cooked ® 1.9 mg 3.5 ounces

* Data from USDA – Iowa State University Database on the Isoflavone Content of Food – 1999.

** Data derived from Protein Technologies International.

® VPP is often used in school lunch programs.

Don't let time take your memories

If you think getting older automatically means your memory goes downhill, think again. A recent study in *The Journal of the American Medical Association* (JAMA) found that cognitive decline is not a normal part of aging for most people. Seventy percent of the study's elderly subjects showed no significant loss of brain function over a 10-year period.

So don't assume that aging takes away your brain power. You can do a lot to keep your brain sharp for the rest of your life — even if you live past 100.

Avoid atherosclerosis. As you get older, your arteries gradually become less flexible, which could affect blood flow to your brain. If you also have built-up fatty deposits in your arteries, you're even more likely to suffer a loss of brain power. The JAMA study found that people with severe atherosclerosis are at a much higher risk for memory loss.

To keep your brain functioning at its peak for years to come, control your risk factors for atherosclerosis now. A high-fat diet, smoking, and a sedentary lifestyle can make you more susceptible to atherosclerosis. So can high blood pressure, high cholesterol levels, and diabetes. Read more about these conditions to learn how to avoid them.

Keep moving. You know exercise is good for your body, but did you know it's also good for your mind? Aerobic exercise may be particularly effective.

One recent study found that small increases in aerobic fitness improved mental fitness, especially functions that control the ability to plan and organize. You don't have to join an aerobics class, either. Study participants engaged in brisk walking as their aerobic exercise.

And a recent study on mice indicated that exercise may even stimulate the growth of new brain neurons, which until recently was not believed to occur in adult mammals.

Break the stress cycle. Cutting stress from your life completely may be an impossible task, but if you value your memories, you should at least try to control your stress level.

Research finds that extreme stress causes your hippocampus to shrink. This is the part of your brain most closely involved with memory. A study of Vietnam vets with post-traumatic stress syndrome found that those who spent more time in combat had significantly smaller hippocampi.

You may not have the stress level of a soldier in combat, but controlling your anxieties may help you hold onto your pleasant memories a little longer.

Feed your brain. Your brain needs nourishment just like your body. A large study of people over age 60 found memory problems in almost 20 percent of those who skipped meals or did not eat enough. Only 7 percent of those who ate regular meals had poor memories.

Get plenty of vitamin E. The same study found that elderly people with low levels of vitamin E were more likely to have poor memories. Foods high in vitamin E include wheat germ oil (and most plant-based oils), peanuts, and mangoes.

Boost your aging brain with blueberries

Time marches on, and there's nothing you can do to stop it, but a new study suggests that something as simple as eating blueberries may help reverse the aging process — at least when it comes to your brain.

In the study, male rats equivalent in age to humans in their 70s were fed plain chow or chow supplemented with extract of either blueberry, strawberry, or spinach. After eight weeks, the four groups of animals were tested on motor function, memory, and cognitive ability.

All three groups of rats that got the supplemented chow did better than the other rats on memory and learning tests. The supplements, especially blueberry, were also effective in preventing age-related declines in brain function and performance. The blueberry-supplemented group did significantly better on tests that measured balance and coordination.

Whether these results would be the same in humans remains to be seen, but researchers think they may, because fruits and vegetables contain antioxidants. Antioxidants fight free radicals, which are harmful chemicals that are created as your body processes oxygen. Your brain may be a particular target for free-radical damage, because it uses so much oxygen — about 20 percent of all the oxygen you inhale.

Other studies suggest the same thing. In a study of more than 5,000 people ages 55 to 95, researchers found that those people whose diets included the most beta carotene (a carotenoid with antioxidant abilities) were the least likely to have problems with memory, attention span, and other mental abilities. Foods high in beta carotene include carrots, spinach, sweet potatoes, and apricots.

Eating blueberries and spinach may not stop the aging process, but it's an easy and delicious way to hedge your bets — and perhaps protect your brain.

• •
Do cell phones cause memory loss?

Ever since cell phones hit the market, people have been concerned about the potential health hazards. Now preliminary research suggests that microwaves similar to those given off by cell phones may affect your memory.

Researchers exposed one group of rats to the same type of radiation cell phones give off and then had them try to find a submerged platform. The rats who were exposed to the microwaves seemed to be more confused and had a much harder time swimming to the platform than rats who were not.

Researchers don't know if humans would be affected the same way. But until they know more, you may want to limit the time you spend on your cell phone — or use a headset — to offset any possible danger.

• •

How fat can protect your memory

Whenever you hear the word "fat" it always sounds like a negative, doesn't it? But there are positive benefits from fat, and one of those may be a better memory — if you eat the right kind of fat.

A recent study in Italy found that a diet high in monounsaturated fatty acids (MUFAs) protects against memory loss and the decline of brain functions often associated with aging.

This could be because monounsaturated fatty acids are part of brain membranes, and researchers say that as people age, their bodies need more unsaturated fatty acids.

The study confirmed earlier findings that a higher education level protected against a decline in brain function with aging. However, it also showed that a high intake of MUFAs helped protect those with a lower education level.

The study took place in Italy where one of the most common MUFAs, olive oil, is a large part of the diet. Researchers examined nearly 300 healthy elderly people who reported eating a typical Mediterranean diet with 17.6 percent of their total calories coming from monounsaturated fatty acids. Olive oil accounted for 85 percent of those MUFAs.

Adding a little olive oil to your diet may be an easy and delicious way to protect your memory, and you may protect yourself from other health problems as well. Studies have found that olive oil may protect against heart disease, diabetes, and arthritis. It is particularly effective at improving cholesterol levels. In fact, adding olive oil to a low-fat diet produces better cholesterol results than just cutting out fat.

Monounsaturated fatty acids can be found in other kinds of oils, too, including sesame, corn, sunflower, soybean, and cottonseed. Just remember that if you add olive oil or other MUFAs to your diet, you need to balance out your fat intake by reducing your intake of saturated fats.

PS — remember to take your 'smart pill'

Wouldn't it be nice if you could just pop a pill and improve your memory? The "smart drug" craze has been trying to cash in on that by formulating supplements to improve your brain power. They may contain vitamins, herbs, hormones, stimulants, amino acids, or fatty acids. Research finds that the most promising substance of all may be phosphatidylserine (PS).

Phosphatidylserine is found naturally in your brain and throughout your body. It is a major building block for nerve cells, and it helps stimulate production of important brain chemicals like acetylcholine, dopamine, and protein-kinase C.

Multiple scientific studies have found that PS consistently benefits memory, learning, concentration, word choice, and other measurements of brain function. It also improves mood and your ability to cope with stress. In Europe, it's often prescribed for Alzheimer's.

While PS may improve your brain, simply taking a pill won't turn a dunce into an Einstein. But so far, results are positive and no serious side effects have been reported.

So is there a catch? Finding pure PS may be difficult if you don't have access to the Internet, although some "brain" formula supplements contain PS, along with gingko or other ingredients. And once you find it, the price may be a little stiff. "Brain Gum" with PS currently costs about $60 for a month's supply.

Save your teeth to save your memory

A recent study found that chewing may help you lose weight. Now researchers find it may also improve your memory.

Scientists pulled molars in some mice so they couldn't chew, then tested them on their ability to find their way to a platform through a water maze. Young mice were able to find the platform easily regardless of whether their molars had been pulled. However, older mice without molars had a much harder time than the older mice that still had all their teeth.

When researchers looked at the brains of the mice, they found a possible explanation — brain cells called glia had deteriorated in the toothless mice. They then used magnetic resonance imaging (MRI) to look at the brains of older people. When the people were chewing, an area of the brain known for processing memories would light up.

One theory is that the act of chewing helps relieve stress, which in turn helps prevent memory loss.

Although this is preliminary evidence, it's another good reason to take care of your teeth. So go ahead and chew on some sugarless gum. It might help you remember where you parked your car the next time you're at the mall.

Motion sickness

Make motion sickness go away

You love seeing new places, but if you suffer from motion sickness, getting there can be a miserable experience. Cars, boats, and airplanes all may become sources of nausea and dizziness — although the problem really starts in your ears.

Your ears contain your body's center of balance, and they perceive physical movement. When your body moves, your ears send signals to your brain telling it about the movement. Motion sickness occurs because your eyes don't perceive motion but your body feels it, so your brain receives conflicting signals. Motion sickness can also occur from the opposite situation — simulator-type rides and wraparound movies — where your eyes perceive motion, but your body doesn't feel it.

Whether you plan to travel by car, plane, or boat, here are some tips for combating motion sickness.

Focus on the horizon. Try to focus on a view outside of your vehicle. If you focus on the horizon, your eye will be able to see the results of the motion your body feels. Looking ahead also helps by letting you anticipate turns and bumps.

Be a considerate driver. While the driver of a car seldom experiences motion sickness, he can make things easier for his passengers by avoiding sharp turns and sudden braking and acceleration whenever possible.

Don't read. Reading a book may make those miles roll by faster, but if you're prone to motion sickness, it's best to leave the novel behind.

Stay on deck. Seasickness is more likely to strike when you're below deck with no view of the water. Try to stay on deck and focus on the horizon.

Keep your head still. When your head moves around, movements of the middle ear may cause motion sickness. To help keep your head and body still, try pushing your head firmly against the headrest. Or use a pillow that conforms to your head and keeps it from moving around.

Breathe deeply. Research finds that taking slow, deep breaths can help combat the symptoms of motion sickness.

Eat light. It's a good idea to have something in your stomach before you begin a trip, but make sure it's a light meal. Eat about three hours before setting off, and avoid dairy products and foods high in protein, salt, or calories.

Avoid odors. Smoke and other strong or disagreeable odors can make your queasiness worse, so ask your traveling partners to refrain from smoking or using strong colognes.

Get fresh air. If you start feeling ill, roll down a window if possible, and get some fresh air.

Stay centered. If you're on a boat, the closer to the center you can stay, the better. Movements are less than they are nearer the edges of the boat. This is also true on an airplane.

Try medication. There are several motion-sickness medications available. You can get injections, patches, and other medications from your doctor, or try over-the-counter antihistamine pills. Most doctors recommend patches because they cause fewer side effects, and the benefits last longer.

Spice it up. Many motion-sickness medications cause side effects, especially drowsiness, so an herbal remedy might be better for you. One study found that ginger-root capsules were more effective than Dramamine in preventing nausea.

Put the pressure on. Although there isn't much scientific evidence to support it, some people believe acupressure may help prevent motion sickness. One study did show that an acupressure band applied to the forearm helped prevent nausea after surgery, so it might also help prevent nausea from motion sickness.

Don't drink and ride. Of course you would never drink and drive, but if you're prone to motion sickness, you shouldn't drink and ride, either. Alcohol directly affects your sense of balance and can make motion sickness much worse.

Mouth problems

6 steps to healthy teeth and gums

Everyone likes a nice smile. If you don't take good care of your teeth, however, you could be giving up more than just a nice smile. You could be endangering your health.

Medical studies have found a surprising link between gum disease and heart disease. Researchers think the germs generated by gum disease get into your bloodstream and damage your heart, although not all scientists agree. Some think that people who don't take care of their teeth just aren't likely to take care of other aspects of their health, either.

Still, one study of almost 10,000 people showed a 25-percent increased risk of heart disease in people with gum disease.

Poor oral health may also raise your risk of stroke. A recent study found that people with severe gum disease were twice as likely to have an ischemic stroke, which is caused by blocked arteries, than people with good oral health.

To avoid these serious conditions and keep your mouth in tip-top shape, follow these six steps.

See your dentist regularly. Regular dental checkups are critical for preventing periodontal disease, which is the most common cause of tooth loss. Periodontal infection starts in your gums but can move into the tissues that hold your teeth in place and spread throughout your bloodstream. Because the early stages of periodontal disease are painless, you might not know you have it until it's too late, so see your dentist once or twice a year.

Brush and floss. Of course you've heard this since you were a kid, but it's so important, it bears repeating. Most dentists recommend soft-bristled toothbrushes, and you should choose a fluoride toothpaste that fights gingivitis as well as plaque. Use waxed or unwaxed dental floss at least once a day to clean between your teeth.

Steer clear of stress. Stress may increase the amount and severity of tooth decay. One recent study found that people with ongoing money worries were 70 percent more likely to have periodontal symptoms.

The good news is that people who used effective methods of coping with their financial problems were no more likely to have gum disease than those with no money strains. So if you have stress in your life, financial or otherwise, find ways to cope and you may save your teeth.

Choose your diet wisely. Choosing nutritious foods is a big part of preventing tooth decay and gum disease. Calcium, vitamin D, vitamin B12, and protein are important building blocks for healthy teeth and gums, so make sure you get plenty of these nutrients. If you're dieting, consider taking a daily multivitamin to ensure you're not missing out nutritionally.

Certain foods may promote tooth decay as well. After eating foods high in sugars or starches, the bacteria that causes plaque will actively attack your teeth for at least 20 minutes, so clean your mouth soon after eating them. This doesn't mean just candy. Fruits, milk, bread, cereals, and some vegetables also contain sugars or starches.

Try to limit between-meal snacks, but if you must snack, choose healthy ones like fruit, raw vegetables, cheese, and yogurt, and brush your teeth afterward.

Drink lots of water. It will help flush the toxins out of your body, rinse bacteria out of your mouth, and stimulate your own production of bacteria-fighting saliva.

Avoid acidic foods, which open up the pores in your tooth enamel and allow stains to discolor your teeth. To make your tea or coffee less acidic, add milk.

Chew sugar-free gum. Saliva rinses food particles from your teeth, which helps protect them from cavities. Chewing increases the amount of saliva you produce.

••••••••••••••••••••••••••••
Indulge your sweet tooth with chocolate

If your sweetheart gives you chocolates this Valentine's Day, don't worry about sinking your teeth into them. According to the Academy of General Dentistry (AGD), chocolate really isn't all that bad for your teeth.

Chocolate contains tannins, compounds that are also found in tea. Tannins help prevent bacteria from sticking to your teeth and gums. The AGD says that studies have shown that eating chocolate may actually suppress cavity development.

Of course, even though chocolate may not be as bad for your teeth as once thought, you should still brush your teeth as soon as possible after eating any sugary food.

Chocolate-flavored toothpaste anyone?
••••••••••••••••••••••••••

Hot tips for beating cold sores

It always seems to happen just before a big social event — especially if you're having your picture taken. An ugly cold sore pops up out of nowhere.

Also known as fever blisters, cold sores are caused by the herpes simplex virus. The virus can lie asleep in a nerve of your face, then wake up to cause an outbreak at a most inconvenient time, often when you're under stress.

Besides being unattractive, cold sores can be painful, so you'd probably do anything to avoid them or get rid of them more quickly. Luckily, there are natural strategies available.

Take lysine. This essential amino acid actually seems to counteract the herpes virus. Lysine is considered essential because it can't be manufactured in your body, so you have to get it in the foods you eat or in supplement form.

In our bodies, lysine plays an important role in the repair of damaged tissue and in the production of antibodies, hormones, and enzymes. Lysine is available in supplements, but if you prefer to get it from natural sources, choose lean red meat, cheese, milk, eggs, fish, lima beans, potatoes, soy products, and yeast.

Avoid arginine. To enjoy the healing properties of lysine, you need to avoid foods that contain the amino acid arginine, which blocks lysine's action. Foods such as peanuts, walnuts, seeds, whole grains, rice, and gelatin are high in arginine. To avoid a cold sore attack, don't eat large servings of these foods, especially before an important occasion.

Try aloe vera. The gel from the aloe vera plant is a time-tested remedy for burns, itchy skin, and poison ivy. It may also help cure mouth sores. Aloe vera has anti-viral and anti-inflammatory properties and also contains skin-healthy amino acids, along with vitamins B1, B2, B6, and C. Apply an aloe vera lip balm three times a day until your cold sore dries up. Some doctors even recommend that you drink aloe vera juice to treat internal mouth sores.

Pop an aspirin. This pain reliever may also relieve your cold sores. After a man with recurrent cold sores began receiving a daily dose of aspirin for a heart condition, he reported that his cold sores disappeared. Then, a study at Semmelweis Medical University in Hungary found that 125 mg of aspirin daily taken at first sign of an outbreak cut healing time in half.

Although these results haven't been proven yet, taking an aspirin shouldn't hurt you unless you're allergic to it. Also, if you have stomach or bleeding problems or are on anticoagulant therapy, ask your doctor before taking aspirin.

●●●●●●●●●●●●●●●●●●●●●●●●●●●
Kiss cavities goodbye

The next time you pucker up for a kiss, you'll enjoy an extra benefit besides the obvious one. You'll help yourself and your kissing partner avoid cavities.

According to the Academy of General Dentistry, kissing helps prevent cavities by increasing the amount of saliva you produce. Saliva is your body's natural cavity fighter because it helps wash away food particles and bacteria. It also contains mineral ions that help repair early tooth enamel erosion.

If you don't have a smooching partner handy, try chewing a stick of sugarless gum — it will increase saliva production three-fold. Or, as anyone on a diet can tell you, just think about food, and your saliva production will rise.

●●●●●●●●●●●●●●●●●●●●●●●●

When bad breath means bad health

If everyone leans back just a little whenever you talk to them, you might have a problem with bad breath. Popping a breath mint once in a while might make your breath more socially acceptable, but sometimes bad breath is an indicator of an underlying health problem.

Up to 90 percent of bad breath originates in your mouth. The most serious dental problems that cause bad breath are periodontitis and tooth abscesses. Both these conditions can cause an unpleasant taste in your mouth and intense pain when chewing on the affected side. See your dentist as soon as possible to avoid tooth loss or an infection in your bloodstream.

The other 10 percent of bad-breath cases could be caused by a medical condition like one of the following:

Chronic kidney failure. If your breath constantly smells fishy or like ammonia, and you have stomach pain, itchy skin, fatigue, paleness, and muscle cramps, along with pain, tingling, and numbness or burning in your legs and feet, you might have chronic kidney failure.

Cirrhosis of the liver. This condition gives your breath a musty, rotten-egg odor. If you have mild jaundice, mental confusion, poor appetite and weight loss, fatigue and weakness, nausea or vomiting of blood, and excess fluid in your legs or abdomen, you could have cirrhosis of the liver. A history of hepatitis, liver damage, or alcohol consumption increases your risk.

Diabetic ketoacidosis. If you are diabetic, fruity-smelling breath could mean you have diabetic ketoacidosis, a dangerous condition in which your glucose level is severely out of balance. Other symptoms include stomach pain and tenderness, weakness, nausea and vomiting, and rapid heartbeat. This is a medical emergency, and you should get help immediately.

Lung condition or infection. A lung abscess, bronchitis, pneumonia, or emphysema can give you bad breath. Watch out for these warning signs — chronic cough with or without sputum, shortness of breath, fever and chills, and weight loss.

Sinus infection. Constant bad breath, sinus drainage, headache, pain around your eyes and cheeks, and a general ill feeling could mean you have a sinus infection.

Sjögren's syndrome. Bad breath caused by extreme dryness of your mouth and nasal passages could indicate Sjögren's syndrome. This autoimmune disease, which is common in people over age 50, can also cause painful joints.

Stomach disorders. Any condition that allows air (and therefore odors) from your stomach to travel up into your mouth can cause bad breath. Gastroesophageal reflux (GERD) is the most common offender. If you only have bad breath occasionally, it may be caused by GERD, which also occurs sporadically.

Trimethylaminuria. This disorder, called fish-odor syndrome, may affect as many as 1 percent of the population. It causes an overall body odor and a "fishy" breath odor. This occurs when your body can't process choline properly, leading to an accumulation of a substance called trimethylamine.

This substance has a fishy odor, which passes out through sweat, urine, saliva, blood, and the air exhaled through the mouth and nostrils. If you have this disorder, limit or eliminate your intake of foods high in choline, such as broccoli, beans, eggs, legumes, kidney, and liver.

Osteoporosis

Eating right — the key to prevention

If you don't know how serious osteoporosis can be, consider these facts — this disease affects about 200 million people worldwide and causes about 1.5 million fractures each year in the U.S. alone.

And these fractures are usually much more serious than the broken arm you may have had when you were seven. Spinal fractures caused by osteoporosis can be extremely painful and can sometimes cause deformity, collapsing your posture severely. It can also be a fatal disease, as 20 percent of women who experience hip fractures caused by osteoporosis die within one year.

The good news is that you can help prevent this "brittle-bone" disease. Start eating right today, and you may avoid a lot of pain in the future.

Start with calcium, of course. By now, everyone should know that calcium is essential for strong bones. It is most important before age 40, so you can build a strong bone foundation. Unfortunately, an estimated 75 percent of females under age 35 get less than 800 mg of calcium daily.

The National Institutes of Health and the National Osteoporosis Foundation recommend up to 1,000 mg of calcium daily for men and premenopausal women and up to 1,500 mg for postmenopausal women. Start today to increase your intake of calcium.

Add some vitamin D. Because vitamin D helps your body absorb calcium, you need it to build strong bones. Good nutritional sources of vitamin D include milk, butter, eggs, fish, and liver. Your body also manufactures vitamin D from sunlight, so getting outside is another good way to boost your bones.

Kick in a little vitamin K. Research is beginning to show that vitamin K may also be important for bone health. One study found that women who had higher intakes of vitamin K were significantly less likely to suffer a hip fracture than women with the lowest vitamin K levels. Good sources of vitamin K include turnip greens, liver, cabbage, cauliflower, and soybean oil.

Toss in some salad. Veggies are good for you in many ways, and one of them is keeping your bones healthy. A recent study found that, in men, every extra serving of fruits or vegetables daily resulted in a 1 percent increase in hip bone density. Each 1 percent increase in bone density translates into a 5 percent lower risk of suffering a fracture.

Serve up soy. People in eastern countries like China and Japan are less likely to develop osteoporosis. Scientists think that could be because soy is a regular part of their diet. Several studies have indicated that including soy protein in your diet can increase your bones' density. Soy protein is rich in bone-building calcium and isoflavones, so try a little tofu, tempeh, or soy milk for a change. (New research claims soy may accelerate brain aging. For more information, see the *Mental impairment* chapter.)

● ●
Better bones from (surprise!) broccoli

Move over milk, there's a new super bone-protecting food in town. A new study has found that the more broccoli you eat, the more protection you'll have from osteoporosis and hip fractures.

The study of more than 1,000 women over age 67 found that those who ate broccoli three or more times a week had about one-fifth the risk of hip fracture of women who ate broccoli less than once a week. The broccoli lovers also suffered less bone loss.

Researchers say that broccoli's high vitamin-K content could be responsible for its bone-protecting qualities. Broccoli is already well-known as a nutritional powerhouse, and this may be one more reason to enjoy it often.

● ●

Making the most of your calcium

Calcium is essential for building healthy bones and avoiding osteoporosis. Milk and other dairy products are most people's main source of calcium. But what if you don't like dairy or can't tolerate it? And even if you get lots of calcium-rich foods in your diet, other substances can cause all that calcium to go straight through your body and right down the drain.

Here are a few tips for getting your calcium and making sure your body uses as much of it as possible.

Vary your diet. If you don't like dairy products, you have other calcium options. Sardines, salmon, beans, and green leafy vegetables have calcium, too.

One leafy green that may not be a good source of calcium, though, is spinach. Although it has calcium, it also contains oxalic acid, which keeps you from absorbing the calcium. So eat your spinach for all the great nutrients it offers, but don't count on it as a source for this important mineral.

Take the best supplement for you. It's usually better to get your vitamins and minerals naturally, but if you don't get enough calcium in your diet, take supplements. Studies show that calcium supplements are also effective at strengthening your bones.

And if you're confused about which one to take, look for those with calcium citrate as the main ingredient. A recent study found that calcium citrate supplements were 2.5 times more absorbable than calcium carbonate supplements.

Space out your intake. Your body only absorbs about 500 mg of calcium at a time, so it's best to get calcium-rich foods at each meal. Most calcium supplements should be taken between meals to get the most benefit.

However, calcium carbonate sometimes causes side effects such as nausea, gas, and constipation, so you're better off taking that type of supplement with meals. Some experts also recommend taking supplements at night because blood calcium levels drop during the night.

Skip the salt shaker. You may love salty foods, but they're not doing your bones much good. Sodium competes with calcium for absorption, so if you eat a lot of salt, calcium may pass through your body without being used.

Can the caffeine. That cup of coffee may help get you moving in the morning, but it may be weakening your bones as well. The caffeine in one cup of coffee can increase your need for calcium by 30 to 50 mg for the day. So if you have to drink that morning cup, at least make sure you add some milk.

Check your medications. Certain drugs can interfere with the way your body absorbs calcium. For example, antacids that contain aluminum hydroxide may cause calcium loss. Ask your doctor or pharmacist whether any medications you're taking might affect your calcium level.

Don't diet your bones away

Losing weight has become a national pastime in the United States. Getting down to a healthy weight is a good thing to do, but be careful. While you're thinning down your body, you may also be thinning down your bones.

Being overweight makes you more likely to develop many diseases, including diabetes, heart disease, and cancer. One disease you're less likely to develop, however, is osteoporosis. It is well-established that heavier women have greater bone mineral density (BMD). A higher BMD means a lower risk of osteoporosis.

While the effect of more weight on osteoporosis risk is established, less is known about the effect of weight *loss* on your bones. But a recent study found that just a small weight loss caused a drop in bone density.

The study compared the bone density of 115 premenopausal women on a low-fat diet with that of 121 non-dieters. Dieters lost an average of 7 pounds. Weight loss was associated with a two-fold loss in hip BMD but not as much in spine BMD.

Researchers have several theories for why this may have occurred. Less weight on your body puts less stress on your bones, affecting the rate at which they rebuild cells. Less fat may affect the amount of estrogen available to your body, which in turn can affect bone density. A weight-control program might also limit the amount of calcium you take in, putting your bones in jeopardy.

If you're overweight, however, don't use osteoporosis as an excuse to keep the weight on. You'll be putting yourself at risk for many other serious conditions. Follow these tips for protecting your bones while achieving a healthy weight.

- If you diet, do so only for health reasons.

- Always make sure you get plenty of calcium, but especially if you're on a weight-loss program. Take supplements if necessary.

- Any good weight-loss program should include exercise. Studies show that moderate aerobic exercise can increase BMD, so concentrate on losing weight from exercise rather than from calorie restriction.

- Make your exercise weight-bearing. Some examples include jogging, aerobics, dancing, and weight lifting. Gardening has also been found to be a good weight-bearing activity.

• •
Yard work builds strong bones

Working in your yard can do more than give you the most beautiful lawn on the block — it could help give you the strongest bones, too.

Exercise, particularly weight-bearing exercise, helps increase bone density. And a recent study found that gardening may be one of the best activities for building bones.

Researchers found that women who gardened at least once a week had higher bone density than women who did other types of exercise like aerobics, jogging, swimming, and walking. The only other activity that gave as much protection as gardening was weight training.

However, gardening is done outdoors, which exposes women to bone-healthy, vitamin D-boosting sunlight. But perhaps even more importantly, most women enjoy gardening. For any exercise to be effective, it has to be continued, and people are more likely to continue an exercise they enjoy.

So get out there and start digging and weeding. Your bones will appreciate it.

• •

6 smart ways to conquer the fear of falling

When you were a child, you probably fell a lot and had the skinned knees and bruises to prove it. As you move into your golden years, you're again more likely to fall, but the results can be much more serious.

Falls are the second leading cause of accidental death in the United States and affect mostly older people. One-third of the people who are hospitalized with a hip fracture from a fall die within a year.

Even if you aren't seriously injured by falling, the fear of falling can affect your quality of life. Many older people who fall become afraid to move around as much. This makes them more likely to fall again because they aren't keeping their muscles in shape or practicing their balance.

Don't let falling, or the fear of it, interfere with your life. Follow these tips for a more sure-footed future.

Try tai chi. Regular exercise is the best way to ensure that you maintain muscle strength and good balance as you age, and tai chi is an ideal choice. Tai chi is an ancient Chinese martial art that has gradually evolved more into a form of relaxation and balance exercise than an active type of self defense.

Research has shown that tai chi can help prevent falls. One study of 200 people ages 70 and older found that people who completed a 15-week tai chi program took about half as many falls as before. The tai chi group also had far fewer falls than other groups who went through high-tech computerized balance training or who received information on preventing falls but no specific training.

Keep items within easy reach. Try not to store things you use frequently in high places. If you have to get something on a high shelf, always use a step stool, never a chair. If possible, get a step stool with handles.

Wear the right shoes. Sensible shoes are a must for good balance. Avoid shoes that are unstable, like high heels and shoes with thick soles. Instead, go for snug, comfortable shoes with laces and rubber soles, and always keep your laces tied.

Take your time. Sitting up too fast or jumping to your feet quickly can cause head rushes and dizziness that could lead to a fall. After sitting up in bed, wait a few seconds on the side of the bed to get your bearings before standing.

Monitor medications. When your doctor prescribes a medication, ask him if it could cause dizziness as a side effect, and if so, whether you could take something else. Also try not to take multiple medications unless necessary.

Fall-proof your home. Take the time to make sure your house is a safe environment.

- **Stairs.** Make sure your staircases have handrails on both sides of the stairs, and cover stairs with tight-knit carpeting or nonslip treads.

- **Rugs.** Ideally, anyone at risk of falling should eliminate throw rugs from their home. If you must have them, however, at least make sure you anchor them with double-sided tape, and try to keep them out of high-traffic areas.

- **Floors.** Shiny waxed floors are pretty but may be dangerous and slippery. Keep muddy shoes, umbrellas, and other items out of high-traffic areas. They're just waiting to be tripped over.

- **Light.** Be sure your home is well-lit, inside and out, particularly in areas of uneven or awkward footing, such as stairs. For security at night, keep a night light burning in the bathroom, the bedroom, and wherever else you may roam.

- **Bathroom.** Use nonslip backing on bathmats and rugs. If your tub is slippery, put down nonslip tape to help you keep your footing. If you have trouble getting up and down, install a handrail in the tub and next to the toilet.

● ●
A cupful of bone protection

If you enjoy a nice cup of tea, you might make your bones stronger — even if you don't add milk to it.

A recent British study found that women who drank tea had greater bone mineral density (BMD) than women who didn't drink tea.

The women were divided into two groups — those who drank tea with milk and those who didn't — to avoid confusing results from the calcium in the milk. Still, tea drinkers who added milk only had higher BMD in one bone area than tea drinkers who didn't add milk.

The protective effect may come from flavonoids found in tea.

This was a preliminary study, so researchers aren't suggesting you swap your milk mug for a teacup, but if you're already a tea drinker, sip away. You could be building stronger bones.

● ●

Top treatments for osteoporosis

Prevention is the best treatment for osteoporosis, but if you have already experienced thinning bones or osteoporosis-related fractures, you need to know your best medical options. Here are some of the treatments that could help you overcome this life-threatening disease.

Estrogen — Estrogen therapy is the most commonly prescribed treatment for osteoporosis. Estrogen is directly involved in bone metabolism and may also help you absorb calcium. Women who begin estrogen replacement therapy within three years of menopause and remain on it for six to nine years lower their risk of fractures of the spine, wrist, and hip by 50 to 70 percent.

Estrogen therapy has its pros and cons. Besides protecting your bones, estrogen can relieve the hot flashes and vaginal dryness that sometimes accompany menopause, reduce mood swings, improve sleep, and lower the risk of Alzheimer's, colon cancer, and heart disease. But it also may cause vaginal bleeding, weight gain, breast tenderness, nausea, and headaches. And some studies have suggested that it could increase your risk of breast or endometrial cancer.

Raloxifene (Evista) — This medicine is a Selective Estrogen Receptor Modulator (SERM). It acts like an estrogen on bone cells but not on breast and uterine tissue. Therefore, it isn't as likely to cause some of the side effects of estrogen replacement therapy, like vaginal bleeding or increased risk of breast or endometrial cancer. It may even protect against breast cancer.

However, it won't help you with other symptoms of menopause like hot flashes, and it may not be as effective on bone mass as estrogen. It may be a good choice for women who want to protect their bones but are concerned about the long-term effects of estrogen therapy.

Alendronate (Fosamax) — This drug is a bisphosphonate, which is a form of a compound that naturally occurs in bone. Studies have found that it increases bone mass and reduces fracture risk, even in older women with previous fractures. One drawback is that you have to take it with water while sitting upright, because it can damage your esophagus if it doesn't pass quickly into your stomach.

Risedronate (Actonel) — In two large studies, this new drug reduced the risk of new spinal fractures by up to 74 percent in post-menopausal women after just one year of treatment. It is the first drug found to affect spinal fracture risk that quickly, so it could be extremely valuable in treating women who have already had spinal fractures.

Calcitonin — This drug is available as an injection and as a nasal spray. It reduces bone loss, but there is less evidence that it helps prevent fractures, so it may not be a good choice for people who have already suffered fractures.

Osteoprotegerin — This natural protein isn't available as a treatment yet, but one large study found that just one shot cut bone loss by 80 percent in postmenopausal women. After a month, however, the women had returned to their pre-shot rate of bone loss, so you would have to get monthly shots for it to be effective.

Many more studies are needed before this drug would be approved, but it may lead to a new and effective way to treat osteoporosis in the future.

● ●
'Bone' up on hormones — it could save your skeleton

Estrogen therapy is one of the leading treatments for osteoporosis, so obviously hormones can affect your bones. However, estrogen isn't the only hormone you need to know about. Your thyroid and parathyroid glands also produce hormones that may affect the health of your bones.

Your thyroid is located in your neck and helps to regulate your metabolism. Sometimes this gland produces too much thyroid hormone (hyperthyroidism) or too little hormone (hypothyroidism). If you've taken drugs to correct these problems, your bones could be suffering the consequences.

Although there is conflicting evidence, some research finds that thyroid-suppressing drugs may contribute to lower bone density. A few other studies suggest that taking additional thyroid hormones may be harmful. If you've taken thyroid-suppressing drugs or thyroid hormones, you should have a bone scan done regularly.

On the other hand, your parathyroid glands may be the key to better bones in later life. These small glands near your thyroid produce parathyroid hormone (PTH), which regulates calcium and phosphorus metabolism.

In a recent study, two-thirds of women with postmenopausal osteoporosis who took parathyroid hormone in addition to their estrogen therapy regained full, healthy bone mass. The women in the study who continued their estrogen therapy without adding parathyroid hormone only experienced a small 1.5 percent gain in bone mass.

If all goes well, parathyroid hormone may soon be available as an osteoporosis treatment. Check with your doctor.

● ● ● ● ● ● ● ● ● ● ● ● ● ● ● ● ● ● ● ●

Ovarian cancer

How to avoid this silent killer

Cancer is much more likely to be treated successfully if it is discovered early. Unfortunately, ovarian cancer is difficult to detect early because it often causes no symptoms until it has spread. And even when symptoms appear, it is easy to ignore them because they're so vague.

These symptoms include a swollen, bloated feeling; discomfort in the lower abdomen; loss of appetite or feeling full after eating just a few bites; and weight loss. You may also experience digestive symptoms, such as gas, indigestion, nausea, diarrhea, constipation, or frequent urination. Occasionally, vaginal bleeding is a symptom of ovarian cancer.

It's important to remember that these symptoms could also be caused by less serious conditions. Make sure you have regular checkups, and tell your doctor if you're experiencing any symptoms. It also doesn't hurt to practice a little prevention. Here are some steps you can take to avoid this life-threatening disease.

Discover the power of antioxidants. A recent study found that what you eat now can affect your future risk of ovarian cancer. Antioxidant-rich green leafy vegetables were most strongly associated with decreased risk. Good choices include spinach, collard and turnip greens, and dark green lettuce.

But green leafy vegetables aren't the only ones that protect against ovarian cancer. Other studies show that beta carotene, an antioxidant found in brightly colored fruits and vegetables, also offer protection, with carrots topping the list.

Another important antioxidant is the mineral selenium. Researchers at Johns Hopkins University in Maryland found that high levels of selenium were associated with a lower risk of ovarian cancer. If you want to improve your odds against this cancer, make sure you eat selenium-rich foods, like seafood, grains, and vegetables.

Limit egg yolks. If you're concerned about ovarian cancer, you might want to eat fewer egg yolks. Researchers suspect a link between cholesterol and ovarian cancer, and egg yolks are high in cholesterol. Egg whites and cholesterol-free egg substitutes are good alternatives to whole eggs.

Go easy on dairy foods. A high intake of lactose, a natural sugar found in dairy products, also increased ovarian cancer risk for some women. But don't limit your dairy intake too much, since it's a good source of calcium.

Pass on the powder. Anything that can cause inflammation of your ovaries increases your risk of ovarian cancer. Ovarian cysts, endometriosis, and an overactive thyroid all increase your risk, but you don't have very much control over those factors. One source of inflammation you do have control over is talc use. Multiple studies have found that the use of talcum powder anywhere on your body increases your risk of ovarian cancer.

Pain, chronic

Drug-free way to soothe pain and relieve tension

A technique discovered by a Shakespearean actor who lived around the turn of the 20th century could help you learn to deal with chronic pain.

When this actor, Frederick Matthias Alexander, developed chronic laryngitis, doctors said there was little besides surgery that could help.

Alexander, however, was determined to help himself. He began studying and changing his own body movements and muscle tension in an effort to reduce the strain on his neck and vocal chords. In the process, he discovered he had been abusing his entire body, as well as his voice. When he began to change the way he moved, his voice returned and his overall health improved.

The method he developed and began teaching to others, called the Alexander Technique, is a way of using your body. Through his approach, you learn how to get rid of harmful tension, stress, strain, pain, fatigue, and depression. These are often hidden causes of many physical problems.

It's not an exercise program but a relearning of habits, both physical and mental, to help you calm your mind; relax your body; and improve your breathing, posture, and balance. You learn how to use your muscles in a more efficient way so you can cope better with daily life. You'll discover the best way to do all kinds of everyday activities, like lie down, get up, stand, walk, run, reach, lift, climb, and drive.

If you want to take responsibility for your own health and well-being, learn the Alexander Technique. Although you can find books on the philosophy and fundamentals of the Alexander Technique at your local bookstore or library, you'll need a teacher in order to fully understand and master this technique.

For help finding instruction in the United States, contact:

North American Society of Teachers of the Alexander Technique

(NASTAT)
P.O. Box 517
Urbana, IL 61801-0517

In Canada:

Canadian Society of Teachers of the Alexander Technique

(CANSTAT)
Box 47025
Apt. 12-555
West 12th Avenue
Vancouver, BC V5Z3XO
Canada

How to sail smoothly through surgery

Surgery can be a frightening and painful experience. If you want to make it as safe and easy as possible, check out your surgeon's credentials, as well as the hospital's success rate for your type of surgery, and consider the following recommendations:

Pass on the potatoes. Different people respond in surprisingly different ways to anesthetics, and doctors now think they know why — it could be what they ate before surgery.

Plants in the nightshade family, which include potatoes, tomatoes, and eggplant, contain compounds called solanaceous glycoalkaloids (SGAs). These substances act as natural insecticides, protecting the plants from attack by animals, insects, and fungi.

Unfortunately, even small amounts of these compounds can cause your body to break down anesthetics and muscle relaxants more slowly — causing the anesthetic to remain in your body longer than it should. Until more is known about this phenomenon, it might be a good idea to eliminate nightshades from your diet for at least a few days prior to surgery.

Check your herbs. Before having surgery, tell your doctor about all the medications you are taking, including herbal remedies. As many as 70 percent of the people using alternative medications don't tell their doctors.

While there have been no major studies done on herbs and surgery interreactions, several herbs may cause a problem. For example, gingko can affect your body's blood-clotting ability, which could cause excessive bleeding during surgery. St. John's wort, a popular herbal treatment for depression, could prolong the effects of anesthesia.

If you know you're going to have surgery, stop taking any herbs a couple of weeks before. If you're scheduled for surgery on short notice, tell your doctor about any herbs you've been taking, or show him the packages so he can read the labels.

Relax with a little music. Believe it or not, listening to relaxing music may improve the outcome of your surgery. A recent study found that relaxation and music, either alone or in combination, reduced postoperative pain.

Pain following surgery is not only uncomfortable it can increase your body's reactions to stress following surgery, interfere with sleep and appetite, and contribute to complications that may prolong your hospital stay.

In the study, one group used a jaw relaxation technique, another group listened to music, and a third group used a combination of music and relaxation. All three groups also had access to pain medication. A control group had only pain medication. The three treatment groups experienced significantly less pain than the group that just received medication.

Ask about acupressure. A study at the Maimonides Medical Center in Brooklyn, N.Y., found that the ancient Chinese practice of acupressure can help reduce nausea and vomiting following surgery.

Researchers applied acupressure cuffs to the forearms of people before surgery. Only 23 percent of the people who wore the cuffs experienced nausea after surgery, while 41 percent of the people who didn't wear the cuffs experienced nausea.

The hospital in which the study was performed now offers the cuff as an option for people having surgery. Ask if your hospital can provide one for you, or check into getting one for yourself. The manufacturer of the cuff used in the study was AcuBand Inc., P.O. Box 355, Little Silver, NJ 07739.

● ●
Pain relief from high-tech food bar

How would you like to eat a tasty food bar to relieve your pain? If your pain is caused by peripheral artery disease (PAD), you may soon be able to do just that.

In a study group of 41 people with PAD, those who ate specially designed food bars twice a day for two weeks were able to walk 66 percent further without pain than before.

The food bars contained a high dose of L-arginine, an amino acid that helps your body produce nitric oxide. Nitric oxide helps blood vessels dilate. People with PAD usually have high levels of another substance that suppresses nitric oxide.

Previous studies indicted that L-arginine supplements helped improve blood flow and reduce pain. However, the pills tasted bitter and could cause stomach irritation. Researchers mixed L-arginine with soy and gave it a vanilla or cranberry coating so it would taste better and be less likely to cause stomach problems.

If you have PAD, ask your doctor about this novel approach to controlling your pain.

● ●

The 'write' way to relieve pain

They say the pen is mightier than the sword, and if you have a chronic medical condition, new research finds that the pen may be as mighty as your medication.

A recent study found that people with chronic asthma or rheumatoid arthritis (RA) experienced improvements in their conditions after spending a total of just one hour writing. What they wrote about, however, made all the difference.

Some of the people in the study were asked to write about the most stressful event of their lives in an emotional, insightful manner, and some were asked to write about a neutral topic — how they planned to spend the rest of their day.

Four months after the writing experiment, asthma participants were evaluated with spirometry, which is a way of measuring the air capacity of the lungs, and people in the RA group were examined by a rheumatologist.

The people with asthma who wrote about stressful events showed improvements in lung function, but the people in the other writing group showed no change.

The people in the RA experimental group also showed improvement — a 28 percent reduction in disease severity. The group who wrote about neutral topics had no change in symptom severity. Overall, 47 percent of the people who wrote about stressful events in their lives experienced improvement in disease.

Although researchers aren't sure why the writing exercise helped, it might be worth a try. Just grab a pen and some paper and start writing.

The danger of pain-relieving magnets

People who have chronic pain are often attracted to alternative methods of pain relief to give their bodies a break from medication. Therapeutic magnets are an increasingly popular method of pain relief.

Although scientific evidence to support the healing power of magnets is promising but skimpy, many people swear the devices relieve their arthritis, back pain, and other painful conditions. While magnets aren't officially approved by the FDA, they haven't been banned and are considered fairly harmless.

On the other hand, if you have a pacemaker or implantable cardioverter defibrillator (ICD), using therapeutic magnets could cause your device to malfunction, according to a recent study. A pacemaker helps regulate the rhythm of your heart, and ICDs are designed to detect heartbeat irregularities and shock your heart back into a normal rhythm.

Researchers say the magnets have to be close to your heart to cause a problem. According to tests done during the study, an inch away affected the devices, potentially causing them to shut off, but 6 inches away seemed safe.

Since most magnets are worn on joints, like knees and elbows, they usually aren't a problem. However, some companies manufacture mattress pads with magnets sewn in for people with back pain. If you have a heart device, sleeping on one of these mattresses could spell trouble — and here's why. Rolling over on your stomach while you are sleeping could shut off your device. And if you have a heart rhythm disturbance, which is common during sleep, your device would fail to correct the problem, a dangerous situation for anyone with heart problems.

Nevertheless, if you know the dangers, magnets can be a safe method of pain control, even for people with heart devices. If you don't have a heart device, there are no known side effects to magnetic therapy, although more studies need to be done.

If you're interested in magnets for your chronic pain, call the North American Academy of Magnetic Therapy (1-800-457-1853) for advice and a list of manufacturers.

Parkinson's disease

Natural help for Parkinson's disease

Parkinson's disease is getting more attention lately because public figures like Muhammad Ali and Michael J. Fox have been diagnosed with the disease.

Parkinson's is a disorder in which your brain cells, or neurons, break down. These neurons produce dopamine, a chemical that helps your brain control your muscle movements. When they die, they no longer make dopamine, and your muscles don't work as well.

Parkinson's usually affects people over the age of 50, but it sometimes strikes people in their 20s. It is a little more common in men than in women.

The early symptoms of Parkinson's disease are general and easy to overlook. At first, you may simply feel tired and weak. Then you may notice that your hands tremble while at rest. Your muscles may begin to feel stiff, you may move more slowly, and you may have trouble keeping your balance. You might notice a change in your speech, or your handwriting may become much smaller.

If you think you may have Parkinson's, see your doctor. He can prescribe medicine that will help you. The most common is Levodopa, or L-dopa, which changes to dopamine in your brain. However, L-dopa becomes less effective the longer you use it, so you should try to delay taking this medication as long as possible.

While there isn't a cure for Parkinson's yet, if you're diagnosed with the disease, you can take steps to help control it naturally.

Exercise. If you've always been an active person, keep up your normal activities as long as you can. If you're a more sedentary person, now is a good time to start getting your muscles in better shape. It could help delay some of the stiffness and fatigue that Parkinson's can cause. Aerobic and strengthening exercises are beneficial, but just taking a walk every day will help. Tai chi is an excellent, gentle form of exercise that may also help improve your balance. Most local recreation centers offer classes in tai chi, as well as other exercise classes. Check with your doctor or therapist for specific programs that fit your needs.

Watch what you eat. Some people with Parkinson's find that certain foods make their symptoms worse. For example, hot, spicy foods may make movement more difficult. Keep track of what you eat, and whether it seems to have any effect on your symptoms.

- **Protein.** Researchers discovered that protein can interfere with the body's absorption of L-dopa. If you are taking L-dopa, limit your protein, and try to get most of it at night, when your medicine doesn't have to be as effective.

- **Fat.** Everyone knows too much fat is bad for you, but a recent study found that a diet high in fat may contribute to Parkinson's disease. While more studies need to be done to confirm the findings, it's still a good idea to limit your intake of fat, especially saturated fat. Saturated fat is found in animal products, like meat, egg yolks, milk, cream, butter, and cheese. Several vegetable fats, such as coconut oil, palm oil, and hydrogenated vegetable oils, are also high in saturated fat.

- **Fiber.** Constipation can be a side effect of Parkinson's, so make sure you get plenty of fiber and drink lots of water. Fruits, vegetables, and whole grains are good sources of fiber.

Join a support group. You may have a caring family, but they can't understand what you're going through the way another person with Parkinson's can. Joining a support group may help keep you from feeling alone and depressed, and you may get some helpful advice on how others deal with the disease. Call your local American Parkinson Disease Association to find a support group near you, or call the national headquarters at 1-800-223-2732.

Try therapy. Different types of therapy are available to people with Parkinson's. Physical therapy may help teach you how to deal with your movement problems and increase your mobility. Some people with Parkinson's have speech difficulties because the muscles in the throat and voice box don't work the way they should. Speech therapy may help you speak more clearly and make your disease less noticeable. Psychological counseling may help you overcome the depression that often accompanies Parkinson's.

• •
Pointing the way to better movement

A new tool may help fight a common symptom of Parkinson's disease — sudden transient freezing. This temporary condition comes on suddenly and causes the muscles to become stiff and unmovable. Laser pointers, the same kind used by teachers to point out hard-to-reach areas of maps, could help alleviate these episodes.

In a recent study, people with Parkinson's used the laser pointers as a visual cue, pointing the light about two feet in front of them in the area where they would step. Researchers recorded how fast they were able to move with and without the laser pointer. When using the laser pointers, they moved 30 percent faster.

While the study was very small — only four people — researchers are encouraged by the results because it could provide an easy, affordable way to improve movement and quality of life for people with Parkinson's.
• •

Pawpaws may cause parkinsonism

Fruit is a healthy, sweet treat, and tropical fruits may be especially tempting on a hot summer day. Unfortunately, some tropical fruits may be linked to a higher rate of Parkinson's-like disorders, research has found.

Guadaloupe, French West Indies has an abnormally high rate of progressive supranuclear palsy (PSP) and atypical parkinsonism. Researchers investigated whether herbal teas and fruits of the Annonaceae family, including custard apple or pawpaw fruit, might be responsible. Previous research had linked compounds found in those fruits to parkinsonism in animals.

The study found that people with PSP and atypical parkinsonism were more than 20 times as likely to have eaten those fruits or herbal teas than healthy people or people with conventional Parkinson's disease.

Specifically, 94 percent of the people with PSP and 100 percent of the people with atypical parkinsonism reported having regularly eaten pawpaw fruit, while only 59 percent of people with conventional Parkinson's regularly ate the fruit.

Pawpaws *(Annona reticulata)* are grown in the United States, primarily in the Eastern half of the country. It is the largest edible fruit native to the U.S. Other fruits in the Annonaceae family include *Annona squamosa,* commonly known as sugar apple or sweetsop, and *Annona muricata,* commonly known as soursop or guanabana.

This study suggests that these fruits may contribute to the development of parkinsonism, but more studies need to be done to confirm the findings.

A jolt of java may ward off Parkinson's

If you need at least one cup of coffee to jump-start your day, you may be protecting yourself from Parkinson's disease.

Exciting new research has found that people who drink coffee may be less likely to develop the disease, and the more you drink, the more your risk goes down.

The study looked at more than 8,000 men over 30 years. Researchers found that men who didn't drink coffee were three to six times more likely to develop Parkinson's disease than coffee-drinkers.

But you don't have to be a coffee lover to take advantage of the beneficial effect. The study found the same results for increasing levels of caffeine, regardless of the source.

Researchers can't be sure it's the caffeine that's responsible for the protective effect. It may be some other aspect of the coffee-drinking personality type. Nevertheless, the discovery of a possible protective factor may spark more studies that will someday lead to a cure.

Prostate disease

Secrets for outsmarting BPH

Webster's defines benign as "causing little or no harm; not malignant." If you have benign prostatic hyperplasia (BPH), your problem is not cancerous. It may not even be very harmful, but as any man with BPH who makes numerous, sometimes useless, trips to the bathroom every day will tell you, it can definitely be a nuisance.

BPH is an enlargement of the prostate gland that occurs mostly in men over 40. About half of all men will have some level of BPH by age 60, and by age 85, it affects 90 percent of men.

BPH causes urinary problems because of the prostate's location — right around the urethra, the tube that carries urine from your bladder out of your body. When your prostate becomes enlarged, it puts the squeeze on your urethra, making it more difficult to urinate.

Although BPH is usually more of a nuisance than a danger, it can lead to more serious problems. When urine can't get through your urethra, it has no place to go but back up into your bladder. There it often stagnates and causes urinary tract and bladder infections. You may also develop painful bladder stones or experience sexual difficulties. Untreated BPH can even lead to kidney damage because of increased pressure on the kidneys or the spread of infection from the bladder to the kidneys.

The treatments for BPH include drugs, like finasteride, or surgical removal of the prostate. But there are also natural alternatives for treating and preventing BPH.

- **Saw palmetto.** In several studies, a concentrated extract of saw palmetto berries was at least as effective as the drug finasteride in treating BPH. One study found that men with BPH who took saw palmetto for three months had more than twice the urine flow of men who took finasteride for a year. About 5 percent of the men taking saw palmetto report side effects, most commonly gastrointestinal symptoms, like nausea, constipation, and diarrhea. About 5 percent of men taking finasteride report serious side effects, like impotence, incontinence, and decreased sexual drive.

- **Pygeum.** The bark of the *pygeum africanum* tree, which grows in Africa, is used to make an extract for treatment of BPH and prostatitis (inflammation of the prostate.) It may be a little less effective than saw palmetto for treatment of BPH symptoms. Yet, according to one study, it may improve sexual performance in some men with prostate disorders.

- **Zinc.** Your prostate gland contains high levels of zinc — as much as 10 times the amount of zinc found in other parts of your body. Study results on whether zinc can help with BPH and its symptoms have been mixed, but some results suggest that it may help. The recommended dietary allowance (RDA) for zinc is 12 to 15 milligrams (mg), but some medical experts suggest taking higher doses for BPH. Check with your doctor before taking more than the RDA. Too much zinc can cause nausea, vomiting, dehydration, restlessness, and anemia.

- **Pumpkin seeds.** In some Middle Eastern countries, men eat a handful of pumpkin seeds daily to prevent BPH. And, according to recent research, this traditional treatment may help. In one study, researchers found that a combination of saw palmetto and pumpkin seed extracts improved urinary flow and reduced nighttime urination, pain during urination, and the number of times daily men needed to urinate. Pumpkin seeds may work because they contain chemicals that block the conversion of testosterone to dihydrotestosterone, which tends to promote prostate enlargement. Pumpkin seeds are also high in zinc.

Preventing prostate cancer

Prostate cancer affects mostly older men, but it's never too early — or too late — to start a prevention program.

Move it. Exercise may help prevent prostate cancer. Researchers studying almost 30,000 men found that those who were active in their jobs were less likely to develop prostate cancer. If your job requires you to sit behind a desk, don't worry. Leisure time activities also lowered the risk of developing the disease. And you don't have to spend a lot of time or money on exercise equipment. Walking was the activity associated with the greatest reduction in prostate cancer risk.

Lose it. If you're overweight, you're more likely to get prostate cancer, particularly if you gain weight after age 50. One study found that men with a body mass index (BMI) greater than 29 have an 80 percent greater risk of developing prostate cancer than men with a BMI of less than 23. (See the BMI chart in the *Weight gain* chapter to find your BMI.)

Cut the fat. Probably the best way to keep your BMI under control is to limit your intake of fat, another risk factor for prostate cancer. Men with the highest fat intake have a 79 percent increased risk of advanced prostate cancer than those with the lowest intake. Try to limit your fat intake to no more than 30 percent of your total calories and reduce your intake of saturated fat to 10 percent or less of your total calories.

Try tomatoes. One of the easiest ways to prevent prostate disease may be to eat more tomato products. Researchers have discovered that tomatoes contain a substance called lycopene that may have a protective effect. A Harvard study found that the risk of prostate cancer was reduced by 45 percent among men who ate at least 10 servings of tomato-based products a week. Foods made with cooked tomato products, like pizza and spaghetti, provide more protection than fresh tomatoes.

Beat it with beta carotene. If you eat lots of brightly colored vegetables and fruits, which are rich in beta carotene, you may be protecting yourself from prostate cancer. A recent study found that men who had the lowest blood levels of beta carotene were 45 percent more likely to develop prostate cancer than men with the highest beta carotene levels. You could be giving yourself a double dose of protection if you eat tomatoes, apricots, and watermelon because they contain both beta carotene and lycopene. Other foods high in beta carotene include carrots, sweet potatoes, pumpkin, spinach, and mangoes.

Add some soy. While you're adding more tomatoes and carrots to your diet, maybe you should throw in a little tofu now and then. Japanese men are five times less likely to die from prostate cancer as American men. The difference could be soy intake. A recent study at Loma Linda University in California found that men who drank soy milk once a day reduced their risk of developing prostate cancer by 70 percent.
(New research claims soy may accelerate brain aging. For more information, see the *Mental impairment* chapter.)

Get the right vitamins. Certain vitamins may be more important to prostate health than others. One study found that vitamin D may make prostate cancer cells less likely to spread. Another study found that prostate deaths were highest where exposure to sunlight was lowest. Your body manufactures vitamin D from sunlight.

A recent study also found that antioxidant vitamins C and E may help prevent prostate cancer. These powerful antioxidants cancel out some of the negative effects male hormones have on prostate cells.

Skip the smokes. Smoking affects more than just your lungs. It also increases your risk of prostate cancer. One study found that men who smoked 20 cigarettes daily were 2.9 times as likely to develop prostate cancer as men who didn't smoke.

• •
Surviving prostate surgery

Surgical removal of your prostate is still considered the most effective way to stop prostate cancer, although other options, like cryosurgery (freezing the cancerous cells) and brachytherapy (implanting radioactive "seeds" in the prostate), are becoming more common.

If you and your doctor decide that surgery is the best way to deal with your prostate cancer, do some research to be sure you come out of your surgery safely and with as few side effects as possible.

- **Choosing a surgeon.** Don't be afraid to "shop around" for a good surgeon. A recent study found that the risks of suffering side effects, like urinary incontinence and impotence, were much lower when the surgeon was experienced. Ask the surgeon how many surgeries like yours he's done.

- **Choosing a hospital.** Busier may mean better when it comes to hospitals. One study found that men who had their surgeries done at hospitals with a high volume of prostate surgeries were able to leave the hospital sooner and were less likely to have complications. The men in the busiest hospitals were up to 43 percent less likely to have serious complications and up to 51 percent less likely to die following surgery.

• •

New twist on PSA

One of the secrets to beating any kind of cancer is to catch it early. Even though prostate cancer is a slow-growing cancer, the earlier it's discovered and treated, the better your chances for survival.

A prostate-specific antigen (PSA) test is one way doctors detect prostate cancer. PSA is a protein made primarily by the prostate. You always have a small amount of PSA in your bloodstream. A large amount can be an indication that cancer is present.

The American Cancer Society recommends an annual PSA screening starting at age 50. Some researchers believe that if every man followed those guidelines, the proportion of localized or potentially curable cancers could be increased from about 40 percent without screening to more than 95 percent.

Despite statistics that imply a benefit in prostate screening, the PSA test is still controversial. The test is expensive and can be inaccurate, failing to detect about one-third of prostate cancers, and sometimes indicating that cancer is present when it is not.

Because of this, some experts argue against routine PSA testing, saying it leads to unnecessary treatments that can have serious side effects.

One reason the PSA test may sometimes be inaccurate could be the stress a person is under when he has the test. A recent study found that men with high-stress levels and not much support in their personal lives were two to three times as likely to have high PSA levels.

It may not be a reliable indicator of cancer, but new research suggests that PSA itself may be an important tool in fighting cancer. A recent study found that PSA may slow the growth of prostate cancer by preventing the formation of new blood vessels that feed cancer cells. Researchers say the presence of large amounts of PSA may be your body's way of fighting off prostate cancer. This could explain why it is typically such a slow-growing cancer.

Previous research has looked for ways to suppress the expression of PSA, but this new study suggests that doctors should instead look for ways to use PSA as a treatment option.

You'll have to make your own decision on whether routine PSA testing is best for you, but be assured that research on PSA will continue.

Raynaud's syndrome

Reducing the pain of Raynaud's

If holding a cold can of soda can quickly become a painful experience, you may have Raynaud's syndrome.

This disorder of the circulatory system involves the way your blood vessels react to cold. When most people are exposed to cold, the blood vessels near the surface of the skin narrow just a little to prevent heat from being released from the blood through the skin.

In people with Raynaud's, this response to cold is exaggerated, resulting in greatly reduced blood flow, especially to the hands and feet. Sometimes blood flow to certain areas is blocked completely.

Because of the reduced blood flow, your skin turns white, then blue, and finally red as blood rushes back into the area. It can cause pain, tingling, and numbness. In the most serious cases, the lack of blood flow can cause tissues to die.

Raynaud's affects about 10 percent of the population, usually women between the ages of 15 and 50. If you work with vibrating machinery, play the piano frequently, or have carpal tunnel syndrome, you're at higher risk. Other conditions, such as atherosclerosis, lupus, or rheumatoid arthritis, may also contribute to the development of Raynaud's.

Although Raynaud's is more of a nuisance than a serious threat to most people, you can take steps to protect yourself and make life a little easier.

Bundle up before going out. Studies show that body temperatures in Raynaud's sufferers drop faster than normal and take longer to warm up again. Always wear a warm coat, hat, gloves, and boots when you are outside in cold weather.

Stay warm indoors, too. Cold drafts or even cold air from air conditioning can trigger Raynaud's symptoms when you're indoors. Protect yourself by wearing socks and shoes or slippers all the time, and keep a sweater or blanket handy.

Get some gloves. Keep a pair of clean winter gloves in the kitchen, near your refrigerator, and slip them on before you take a package of frozen food from the freezer or fruit from the vegetable drawer.

Use a "coozie." Insulated foam bottle and can holders will help keep your drinks cold and your hands warm. Or wrap a paper towel around your drinks to insulate your hands from the cold.

Stay away from smoke. If you want to control your Raynaud's, don't smoke and avoid being around people who do. Cigarette smoke takes much-needed oxygen from your body and narrows your blood vessels, making your symptoms even worse.

Try some ginkgo. Ginkgo is an ancient herbal remedy for improving circulation. It may widen your blood vessels, which can improve blood flow in your fingers and toes. You can buy ginkgo in pill form in health food and discount stores.

Move more. Don't sit in the same position for long periods of time. Moving around and exercising regularly helps your blood flow better.

Ditch the caffeine. Caffeine constricts blood vessels, which interferes with circulation. Besides limiting coffee, watch out for caffeine in tea, chocolate, cola drinks, and many cold and cough remedies that contain decongestants.

Keep stress under control. Tension can trigger symptoms even when you're not cold. By finding ways to relax and handle stress, your Raynaud's may improve, too.

Consider hormones. If you take estrogen and have developed Raynaud's, there may be a connection. A recent study found that women taking estrogen were much more likely to develop Raynaud's than those who weren't taking it, or those taking estrogen plus progesterone. If you take estrogen by itself, check with your doctor to see if changing your hormone prescription might help your Raynaud's symptoms.

Try biofeedback. This is a conditioning exercise in which your mind trains your body to keep the blood vessels in your hands and feet open when they should be. You can learn to "think" your fingers and toes warm. Check with your doctor to find someone who can teach you this technique.

Use lukewarm water. If you've been out in the cold weather and want to wash your hands when you come inside, use lukewarm water — hot or cold water may hurt.

Eat an orange. If you have Raynaud's, recent studies suggest you may need more vitamin C and selenium, a mineral found in unprocessed foods. Without these two important nutrients, you are more apt to suffer irreversible tissue damage. Try eating lots of citrus fruits, cantaloupe, strawberries, peppers, papayas, mangos, vegetables and grains, and organ meats, like liver, or take a multivitamin/mineral supplement.

Rub on some gel. A recent study in Great Britain found that a gel containing nitric oxide improved blood circulation in the forearms and fingers of people with Raynaud's. Nitric oxide is a body chemical that helps control blood flow by causing blood vessels to expand. Ask your doctor if this gel is available in your area.

Ask your doctor about *H. pylori.* A recent study uncovered a connection between Raynaud's and H. pylori, the bacterium that can cause ulcers. A group of people who had both Raynaud's and an H. pylori infection were given therapy for a week to get rid of the bacteria. Surprisingly, Raynaud's symptoms disappeared completely in 17 percent of the people who were cured of the H. pylori infection. Among the people who still had Raynaud's, 72 percent experienced fewer and milder attacks. Ask your doctor if a simple antibiotic is the answer you've been looking for.

Respiratory ailments

Avoid talc for healthy lungs

When an otherwise healthy, nonsmoking, 34-year-old accountant went to a hospital in Belgium complaining of a cough and breathlessness during exercise, doctors were puzzled. They were also very concerned when his chest X-rays showed some patchy areas in his lungs. After learning that he was an amateur magician, the doctors were able to solve the mystery.

As part of his act, he blew up balloons and made figures out of them. The balloons were coated with talc, and since he blew up approximately 150,000 of them a year, he had inhaled enough talc to develop talcosis.

Talcosis usually only affects factory workers who are exposed to large amounts of talc, most often in rubber factories. One woman developed lung disease 40 years after she worked for five years in a factory making rubber hoses. Doctors attributed her disease to high exposure to talc during those years.

The everyday use of talc can also cause problems. Babies and small children are in danger of a severe and often fatal reaction from inhaling talc-based baby powder.

And you may not have to inhale talc to experience its bad effects. The use of products containing talc has been implicated in an increased risk of ovarian cancer. A recent study found that women who use powder in their genital areas are 60 percent more likely to develop ovarian cancer than women who don't use powder, or use it only in other areas.

The chance that you will experience problems with talc is small, but if you must use powder, cornstarch is a healthier choice.

● ●

Add years to your life

Do you want to quit smoking, but you're having trouble making a serious attempt? Maybe a little incentive will help. A recent study found that every cigarette a man smokes takes 11 minutes off his life.

Quitting is no easy task, but your doctor can help. Nicotine patches and prescription drugs are very effective for most people, but you have to make the choice to quit.

The next time you want to buy a pack of cigarettes, consider this. If you resist the urge, you'll save money, but more importantly, you may buy yourself almost two more hours of living.

● ●

Beware of hidden danger in candlelight

Did you know you could expose your family to lead if you burn candles in your home? Some candlewicks contain a metal core to make them stand up better and sometimes that core contains lead.

A recent study at the University of Michigan School of Public Health tested candles by burning them in a 12-by-12 foot enclosed room. After one hour, five out of the 15 brands of candles tested emitted lead levels above the U.S. Environmental Safety Administration's recommendations. The candles used in the study came from China, Mexico, and the United States.

The National Candle Association supports a ban on lead wicks. The organization says its members voluntarily agreed to stop using lead in their wicks, even though there are currently no regulations against lead wicks. Because 95 percent of candles manufactured in the United States are made by members of the association, the greatest risk is from imported candles.

Candle makers aren't required to list ingredients on their products, but if you want to know if a candlewick contains lead, rub a piece of white paper over the unburned wick. If it leaves a gray mark, like a pencil mark, it contains lead.

● ●
Protect your lungs at the pool

Being a lifeguard may seem appealing, but it isn't without its hazards. One unusual risk is "lifeguard lung."

In a recent study, researchers examined people who worked at an indoor pool that featured spraying water. Pool employees experienced two outbreaks of a lung inflammation. After the first outbreak, the pool's ventilation system was altered. Prior to the alterations, 27 percent of the employees experienced problems, but after the alterations, 65 percent were having problems. Symptoms included cough, chest tightness, breathing difficulties, and fever.

Most of the lifeguards recovered after leaving the pool, but some had more persistent problems.

If you work or swim at an indoor pool with a water spray, ask the management if the ventilation system is adequate, or wait until summer and do your swimming outdoors.
● ●

Sinusitis

Simple relief for sinus problems

A recent study found that people with chronic sinus problems experience more pain and less pleasure in their daily activities than people with many other chronic medical conditions.

Consider these natural ways to soothe your sinuses.

Get the right amount of sleep. Not getting enough sleep can make your sinus problems more painful and longer-lasting, but too much sleep can have the same effect. Try sleeping with your head slightly raised to help your sinuses drain at night, or if one side is stuffier than the other, sleep with that side tilted down.

Try exercising. For many people, mild to vigorous exercise opens up nasal passages and clears their breathing. Others find it makes their clogged sinuses worse. Get some exercise and see what works for you.

Keep your air moist. Use a humidifier in your home to put moisture back into the air and make it easier to breathe. It will help keep your sinuses from drying out.

Steam away pain. Some people get relief by placing warm, water-soaked towels directly over their sinuses, holding their face over a steaming sink, or simply breathing in the steam from a cup of hot water. For an extra boost, consider adding pine oil, eucalyptus, or menthol to the water.

Eat foods that help. Some foods can help clear your sinuses. Horseradish, garlic, and cayenne are famous for cutting through tough sinus blockages. Add some to soups or other favorite foods for quick relief. Certain foods can cause stuffiness in some people. Almost any food can be an allergen, but some common culprits are wheat, milk, and red wine. Pay attention to your diet, and don't eat foods that cause problems for your sinuses.

Rinse instead of spray. Over-the-counter sinus sprays provide temporary relief, but if you use them for too long, they can worsen your sinus problems. If you decide to use a nasal spray, don't share it with anyone and discard old sprays. A better alternative may be a nasal rinse you can make at home. Simply mix a half teaspoon of ordinary table salt with 8 ounces of warm water. With a bulb syringe, squirt the solution into your nose and let it soothe and rinse your sinuses.

Press away pain. Some people get relief through acupressure. To try it, apply a few seconds of direct pressure to the inner edges of your eyebrows, the sides of your nose, and the bones below and around your eyes.

If you have a nosebleed as a side effect of sinusitis, don't try to stop it with cotton. The cotton fibers will stick and when you try to pull it out, your nose may bleed again. Instead, pack your nose with a piece of gauze coated with petroleum jelly, and then pinch the fleshy part of your nose right between your eyes for about five to 10 minutes.

If home remedies fail and your infection gets worse, see your doctor before it causes lasting damage.

• •
New twist on sinus infections

If you have one sinus infection after another, and antibiotics don't help, here's good news. Long-lasting relief may be on the way.

A recent study found that most cases of chronic sinusitis are caused by an immune reaction to fungus. The study, which used new methods of collecting and testing mucus from the nose, discovered fungus in 96 percent of the volunteers' mucus. Before this study, no one knew what caused chronic sinusitis.

Antibiotics are effective against acute (short-term) sinusitis, which is caused by bacteria. Scientists say the reason antibiotics are ineffective against chronic sinusitis is because they are designed to combat bacteria — not fungi.

Now that researchers know what causes chronic sinusitis, they can find new ways to treat the condition. Check with your doctor for the latest update.

•••••••••••••••••••••••

Skin problems

Anti-aging nutrients for healthy skin

Do you know what organ is your largest? Here's a hint — it's also your most attractive organ. It's your skin, and like any other organ, you need to take good care of it.

These nutrients are very important for maintaining healthy, younger-looking skin.

Vitamin A. Your skin is more than just pretty packaging. It also serves as a barrier to infections that could invade your body. Vitamin A helps maintain the cells that form this skin barricade. If your cells can't get enough vitamin A, some of them are replaced by cells that secrete keratin. This is the substance that makes your hair and fingernails tough. It also makes your skin dry, hard, and cracked, which increases your chances of infection.

Vitamin A is found only in foods of animal origin, like meat and dairy products. If you'd rather get vitamin A from fruits and vegetables, choose brightly colored varieties, like carrots, sweet potatoes, spinach, cantaloupe, apricots, and broccoli. They are rich in beta carotene, which is converted into vitamin A in your body.

And, if you have a problem with acne or wrinkles, vitamin A products like Retin-A may help. They are available in cream form to apply directly to the skin.

Niacin. Niacin deficiency causes a disease called pellagra, meaning "rough skin." Without this B vitamin, you can develop the red, rough skin that gives pellagra its name. Plenty of skin-saving niacin can be found in meats, including fish and chicken.

And your body converts tryptophan, which is found in almost all proteins, into niacin. Since most people get plenty of protein in their diets, niacin deficiency is uncommon today. Talk with your doctor before taking niacin supplements. High doses of certain forms of this vitamin can cause flushing, itching, rash, and abdominal pain.

Vitamin C. If you want your skin to look fresh and young, instead of dry and saggy, get plenty of vitamin C in your diet. Good sources include sweet red peppers, citrus fruits, green peppers, and strawberries. Vitamin C helps make and maintain collagen, which forms the basis of connective tissue in your body, including skin. Collagen forms scar tissue, which helps heal wounds and burns and supports tiny blood vessels to prevent bruises.

Water. While you're eating healthful, vitamin-packed foods for better skin, wash them down with a tall glass of water. Water works its own moisturizing magic on your skin and teams up with vitamins to help keep your skin soft and smooth.

Top tips for great skin

If you want soft, smooth skin with fewer wrinkles, try these simple tips:

Keep it cool. Wash with warm or cool water. Hot water is too harsh and drying.

Bathe in softness. Baths are less drying to your skin than showers — as long as you use warm water and don't soak longer than 10 minutes.

Take a break. Try to bathe every other day or even just a few times a week. This will reduce the amount of protective oil stripped from your skin.

Make it mild. Use mild soap, particularly on your face. Harsh, deodorant soaps can strip your face of protective oils and may actually contribute to acne. Save the strong, antibacterial deodorant soaps for your underarms, feet, and genital area.

Stop scrubbing. Don't rub your skin too hard in the shower or bath. Vigorous scrubbing can break open the skin and alter its protective barrier. Dry yourself by gently patting or blotting with a soft towel.

Moisturize. Pat on some lotion right after your bath or shower to lock in moisture. Lotions containing petrolatum, a thick, jelly-like substance made from petroleum, are considered by many dermatologists to be the most effective moisturizer. Petrolatum has been proven to reduce the amount of water lost from your skin by about 50 percent. In addition, it protects your skin from irritants and is more deeply absorbed than other moisturizers.

Avoid the elements. Although sunscreen offers some protection from the sun's damaging rays, the best way to avoid weather damage is to limit your skin's exposure to sun, wind, and cold as much as possible.

Go tropical. Avoid dry air. Keep a humidifier running in your home or office.

Don't forget your fingers. Wear gloves when you do housework or dishes to protect your hands from drying chemicals and hot water.

Sleep on your back. It may sound silly, but sleeping on the side of your face can contribute to wrinkles over time. The weight of your head on your pillow can push your skin into folds and wrinkles that could start to become permanent.

• •
Safe and easy way to tan

You like the golden glow of a suntan, but you know that, although a tan may *look* healthy, it's really not. The process that produces the tan actually damages your skin and increases your risk of skin cancer. So how can you achieve a golden glow without sacrificing your skin's health? Sunless tanning lotions may be your answer.

The active ingredient in sunless tanning lotions is dihydroxyacetone (DHA). DHA works on dead cells found on your skin's surface to produce a tan. The color fades gradually and naturally within a few days as the dead skin cells are sloughed off.

Other products on the market that claim to be tanning aids may not work as well as products containing DHA, so read labels carefully.

Self-tanning lotions are easy to use and work well, but the really good news is that they are safe. While tans produced by the sun or by tanning beds damage your skin, the color produced by sunless tanning lotions causes no damage, according to the American Academy of Dermatology.

Tan-in-a-bottle may be the best thing to happen to your skin since baby lotion.
• •

Secrets for a glowing complexion

If you're tired of spending money on skin care products, try these inexpensive, natural skin soothers. The ingredients are everyday items you probably have in your kitchen.

Eggs. You can make a quick and effective facial mask with nothing more sophisticated than an egg white. Just beat one egg white until it's frothy and apply it to clean skin. Let it dry — then rinse. It will tighten your skin like a mini-facelift as it dries.

Mayonnaise. Apply whole-egg mayo to your face and leave it on for 20 minutes. Wipe off the excess with a tissue and rinse with cool water. This mask is great for dry skin.

Cornmeal. Mix cornmeal or oatmeal with enough water to make a thick paste. Carefully apply it to your face with your fingertips and massage gently. This will help remove dry skin and blackheads, and it will tighten your skin as it dries. Rinse well.

Potatoes. You may be able to help clear up facial breakouts and blackheads with a peeled slice of potato — just rub it gently over freshly washed skin. Or, to make your own facial mask for oily skin, cook one large potato, peel, and mash. Mix it with one egg white, a half teaspoon of lemon juice, and two tablespoons of milk to form a smooth paste. Spread it over your face, avoiding the eye area. Leave it on for 15 to 20 minutes, then remove with warm water.

Tea. If you wake up with puffy bags under your eyes, brew yourself a pot of chamomile tea. Chamomile is a naturally soothing herb that temporarily decreases puffiness. Just ice the tea, soak a couple of gauze pads, and place them over your eyes. Byebye bags.

Honey. Make a mask by blending a half teaspoon of honey with a half cup of sliced cucumber to a fine consistency, then spread it over your face. Keep the mask on for about a half hour and rinse. Or mix honey, oatmeal, and lemon juice in a bowl. Use enough to make a thick paste that will stick to your skin. Leave it on your face for about 10 minutes, then rinse. This mask is particularly good for oily skin.

Berries. For a facial with a soothing scent, try spreading mashed strawberries or raspberries over your face.

Milk. For soft skin, try Cleopatra's beauty secret — add four cups of milk to your warm bath water and luxuriate for 15 minutes. Or try adding a cup or two of powdered milk. You'll feel like a queen.

Baking soda. For a simple, inexpensive way to soften your skin, add a half cup of baking soda to your bath water and enjoy.

Protect yourself from poisonous plants

"Leaves of three, let it be" is an old saying to help you identify poison ivy, but don't count on it to help you with other poisonous plants, like poison oak or sumac. Sometimes the leaves of these plants grow in groups of five, seven, or even nine, depending on the environment.

There's another way to identify these plants. Poison ivy has yellow-green flowers and white berries and grows as a low shrub or a vine that climbs up trees. Poison oak grows as a small tree or shrub with clusters of yellow berries and leaves that resemble oak leaves.

The sap in these plants contains urushiol, a substance that causes an allergic reaction in some people. If the plant is damaged even a little, the urushiol resin can get on your skin or clothing and set off a reaction. Urushiol can also stick to pets, garden tools, or other objects and get on your skin.

Consider these skin-saving tips before you head for the great outdoors:

- Wear long sleeves and long pants. If you're going to be pulling weeds, wear heavy-duty vinyl gloves. The resin may be able to penetrate rubber (latex) gloves. Even dead plants can contain the active resin and should not be handled without protection.

- Try a barrier cream. Although most skin creams designed to protect against poison ivy don't work very well, studies find that a product containing 5 percent quaternium-18 bentonite (IvyBlock lotion) is effective in preventing or reducing reactions to poison ivy or poison oak exposure. Another study found three creams to be partially effective — Hollister moisture barrier skin ointment, Hydropel protective barrier ointment, and Stokogard outdoor cream.

- Don't use a string trimmer or mow poisonous plants without a catcher.

- Clean clothing, shoes, and tools that may have come into contact with poison ivy. Wash up with soap and water as soon as you're back indoors.

If you come into contact with a poisonous plant in spite of these precautions, here's what you can do:

- Swab the infected area with alcohol. This helps remove the resin up to 30 minutes after exposure. If you are sensitive to urushiol and you don't clean your skin quickly, redness and swelling will begin in 12 to 48 hours, along with blisters and severe itching. After a few days, your rash will become crusty and scaly, and you should be completely healed in 14 to 20 days.

- Resist the urge to scratch if you can. Scratching will not spread your rash, but your fingernails may carry germs that could set off an infection. You can relieve the itching by soaking in a cool bath or applying wet compresses to the affected area. Taking an antihistamine or trying an over-the-counter hydrocortisone cream can also help. If you have a severe reaction, your doctor may prescribe steroid creams or pills. Calamine lotion can soothe itching and absorb oozing from blisters, but don't use it once the blisters stop oozing and dry up.

- For more relief, drain your blisters. Here's how — insert a needle into the edge of the blister. Gently press the top of the blister to remove the fluid. Hold a piece of tissue or gauze onto the skin to absorb the liquid. Wash the skin well and put on your anti-itch cream, but don't remove the skin covering the blister. This skin protects the delicate layer of skin underneath. And don't open any blisters on your face or genitals. Let your doctor take care of those.

• •
Get a grip on blisters

If you have a long day of hard, physical labor ahead of you, here's a good way to toughen your hands and prevent blisters. Rub them with denatured alcohol three times a day for several weeks before your scheduled appointment with hard labor. Wearing soft, thick gloves and changing your grip can help, too.

• •

Sleep difficulties

Natural solutions for sleepless nights

If you've been tossing and turning more than you've been snoozing lately, you may be tempted to reach for some over-the-counter sleeping pills. Before you do, try these natural solutions.

Stick to a schedule. If you have a regular time to settle down for the night, you'll establish a rhythm to help trigger sleep. Try to get up at the same time every morning, too, even on weekends.

Take time to relax before bed. Take about 30 minutes before bedtime to relax and wind down. Read a good book, take a warm bath, or work on a hobby. Low lights and soft music can help get you in the mood for sleep. Try to avoid watching intense television shows or dealing with unpleasant tasks during your wind-down time. That way you'll be calm, cool, and collected when you get into bed.

Create a comfortable atmosphere. It's much easier to fall asleep if you're comfortable. Start with a good mattress and pillow and wear comfortable clothes to bed. Make sure your room is quiet and dark and keep the temperature at whatever is most comfortable for you.

Don't push it. You can't force yourself to sleep. If you've been lying in bed staring at the ceiling for more than a half hour, get up. Try to do some quiet activities, and then go back to bed. Repeat this as often as needed.

Use your bed for sleep only. Going to bed should signal your body that it's time to sleep. If you watch television, work, or eat in bed, your body may get confused and won't automatically relax for sleep like it should. Of course, sex in bed is OK, and it may even help you relax and fall sleep.

Warm your toes. If you have cold hands and feet, you might benefit from using a hot water bottle or wearing socks on your feet when you first go to bed. Warming your hands and feet and then removing the socks or hot water bottle helps your blood vessels dilate. Research indicates that blood vessel dilation in your feet and hands is an important step in falling asleep.

Exercise. About 20 to 30 minutes of exercise three or four days a week could improve your snooze time — but timing is important. Exercise too close to bedtime can be stimulating rather than relaxing.

Take a bath. Soaking in a warm bath can be very relaxing. A recent study found that elderly people who took a bath before bedtime fell asleep faster and slept better.

Work wonders with warm milk. Warm milk has been a home remedy for insomnia for years. Milk contains tryptophan, an amino acid that researchers say can help you sleep. It's also high in calcium and magnesium, two minerals that are important in producing melatonin, which controls your sleep cycle.

Give up caffeine and nicotine. If you depend on coffee to wake you up in the morning, remember it can also keep you up at night. Limit your intake of coffee, tea, colas, and other drinks containing caffeine, especially in the evening. Caffeine keeps you awake because it's a stimulant, but you may not realize that nicotine in cigarettes is a stimulant, too. If you smoke, don't do it before bedtime.

Ditch the alcohol. You may think that a beer or a glass of wine before bed will relax you and help you fall asleep. It may — but it usually results in wakefulness later on in the night. If you really want to sleep tight, don't drink alcohol in the evening.

Get some morning sun. You'll sleep better at night if you soak up some bright light early in the day. Morning sunshine increases the level of melatonin in your body. This hormone helps regulate your sleep cycle naturally.

Keep your tummy content. Going to bed hungry can keep you awake, but eating a heavy meal before bedtime isn't a good idea either. A busy digestive system can really interfere with peaceful sleep.

Try valerian. This herb has been used for over 1,000 years as a mild sedative and sleep aid. It is particularly popular in Europe, and the German Commission E has approved it as a calmative and sleep-promoting product. Valerian does not interact with alcohol, and it's remarkably free of side effects. For a relaxing cup of valerian tea, add two teaspoons of dried root to a cup of hot water.

Practice gradual relaxation. If you are too tense to sleep, try relaxing your muscles, one group at a time. Beginning with your toes, work your way up — feet, calves, thighs, abdomen, hips, and so forth — until you reach your scalp. By that point, you should be relaxed and ready for sleep.

• •
Why you need 8 hours of sleep

Not everyone needs the same amount of sleep, but most adults need at least eight hours every night to function their best.

When you get an hour less than you need one night, and two hours less than you need the next night, that loss adds up and your body craves those extra hours of sleep.

A sleepy person is more likely to make mistakes and have slower reaction times. According to National Highway Traffic Safety Administration, drowsy drivers cause at least 100,000 crashes in the United States each year.

Although you can catch up on sleep and feel better, research finds that you may be doing your body long-term damage. In a recent study, 11 young men slept only four hours a night for six nights. This lack of sleep affected their carbohydrate metabolism and stress hormone levels.

Decreased carbohydrate metabolism may increase your risk of developing insulin resistance, obesity, and high blood pressure. And high evening levels of the stress hormone cortisol may contribute to the development of insulin resistance and memory problems as you get older.

Other studies have found that sleepless nights can increase your blood pressure and other risk factors for heart disease.

Discover the power of napping

A little catnap in the afternoon can be refreshing, and it can even make you more alert. That's why "power napping" is becoming a trend among some leading corporations in the United States.

Studies have shown that naps can improve performance and increase alertness — for as long as 10 hours after a one- or two-hour nap and six hours after a 45-minute nap.

In a NASA study of airline pilots, those who took short naps during long flights were much more alert and performed better than those who didn't.

Because of studies like these, some corporations are adding "nap rooms" to their facilities to get better productivity from their employees.

Although it's well-established that naps increase productivity, sleep inertia, a grogginess and confusion after awakening, may cause impaired performance in the first few minutes after a nap. But the solution is simple — allow yourself a few minutes to fully awaken before you plunge back into work.

Naps can also interfere with your nighttime sleep patterns. Some people adapt well to a nap in the afternoon, while others experience more sleeplessness at night because of it. Try napping and see if it increases your performance without interfering with your nighttime rest.

Of course, if you work at a company without a favorable napping policy, your afternoon nap could interfere with your employment. Before you drift off to sleep, you better talk with your boss.

● ●
Better sleep = better waistline

Don't have the energy to do endless sit-ups and crunches to flatten your jelly belly? Maybe what you really need is a good night's sleep.

According to a recent study, people treated for sleep apnea (a disorder in which you stop breathing for brief periods during sleep) lost abdominal fat, although they didn't necessarily lose weight. Volunteers not treated for their apnea had no change in fat distribution.

The researchers think it's possible the people lost fat because more sleep altered their metabolism favorably. Or it could be they simply had more energy to burn fat during the day after a good night's sleep.

Either way, if you suffer from sleep apnea, or anything else that could be interfering with your sleep, get it treated. You'll gain a good night's sleep and perhaps lose some inches around your middle.

● ●

Don't let jet lag spoil your vacation

Whenever you cross several time zones, you run the risk of suffering jet lag symptoms, like insomnia, agitation, poor concentration, and fatigue. These symptoms are caused by a disruption in your biological clock.

Your body runs on a 24-hour cycle called circadian rhythms. Your circadian rhythms, which are affected by exposure to sunlight, help your body know when to sleep and when to wake up. Whenever you travel to a new time zone, your circadian rhythms are slow to adjust and remain on their original schedule for a few days. That means your body may want to sleep in the middle of the afternoon, or you may be wide awake at 2 a.m.

You don't have to let jet lag interfere with your fun. Take these steps to help prevent it.

Adjust your schedule. A few days before leaving on your trip, begin to adjust your sleep schedule gradually. The goal is to go to bed an hour earlier or later for each time zone crossed, depending on the direction you're going.

Pick the right arrival time. Choose a flight that arrives in early evening and stay up until 10 p.m. local time.

Stay awake in the daytime. Try to stay awake all day, but if you have to nap, make sure it's no more than two hours.

Eat when the natives do. Getting your body on the local time schedule is the key. Eating at about the same time everyone else does will help.

Don't eat too much. When your body is trying to adjust to a new schedule, don't make it work hard by digesting a lot of food. Try to eat lightly at first by choosing a snack instead of a heavy meal.

Skip the caffeine and alcohol. Avoid caffeine and alcohol right before bedtime. They both can interfere with your sleep.

Exercise. Getting some light exercise during the day should help you sleep at night, but avoid strenuous exercise right before bedtime.

Soak up some sun. Sunlight helps readjust your biological clock, so get outside and soak up some rays.

Drink plenty of fluids. Don't take a chance on becoming dehydrated, especially if you've traveled to a higher elevation. Make sure you drink plenty of fluids.

Try some melatonin. Melatonin supplements may help fight the effects of jet lag. In one study, people who traveled across eight time zones had less jet lag if they took 5 milligrams (mg) of melatonin daily, starting three days before they left home.

Stress and anxiety

5 ways to relieve stress and zap anxiety

In times of danger, anxiety can keep you alert — and maybe alive. But overreacting to everyday stresses can harm your health.

When you're threatened, your body releases adrenaline and cortisol, hormones that prepare you to cope with the problem or run from it. Scientists call this the "fight or flight response."

Nature has provided these life-saving responses for emergency situations. Unfortunately, your body responds the same way to chronic stress — the long-term stress you experience every day. Here's how it affects your health:

- **Weakens bones.** Studies show that exposure to cortisol causes bones to lose mass and become brittle. People who are depressed are more likely to have osteoporosis because their bloodstreams are full of cortisol.

- **Bulks up your waistline.** Both cortisol and adrenaline cause your body to redistribute excess fat to your tummy, which increases your risk of heart disease.

- **Taxes your brain.** Learning to relax will help you maintain brain power. A recent study found that people who were given cortisol for several days to mimic a stressful situation didn't perform as well on memory tests as they had before taking the cortisol.

- **Lowers immunity.** Recent studies prove that stress slows the body's production of natural bacteria and virus fighters. Without the right amount of these germ busters in your body, you go to war against disease without any weapons.

Worried that all your worrying is making you sick? Here are some good ways to relieve stress and keep yourself healthy.

Take a hike. Research confirms that exercise is a great stress reliever. One recent study found that college students who exercised less frequently during periods of high stress had 21 percent more anxiety and 37 percent more physical symptoms than those who exercised more often. This strategy may be especially effective if you find an exercise you enjoy. So take dance lessons, drag that bicycle out of the attic, go for a hike, or get out in your garden. The important thing is to get moving.

Get a pet. Furry friends may keep stress levels on a more even keel. A recent study focused on stockbrokers with high blood pressure. Researchers discovered that when exposed to stressful situations, like an irate client, the stockbrokers who had pets nearby were less likely to experience a significant rise in their blood pressure.

Write it down. Keeping a journal can be very therapeutic, but what you write about may make a difference. Researchers studying people with asthma or rheumatoid arthritis asked them to write about their "most stressful event," while others simply wrote about their daily schedule. Almost half the people who wrote about their most stressful times showed significant improvement, but less than 25 percent of the other people improved.

Try some kava. A plant that grows in the South Pacific may provide stress relief during tough times. Kava has been used for centuries in traditional island ceremonies and acts as a mild tranquilizer. Kava products relax muscles and lessen nervousness and depression. You can find Kava in herb shops and the herb section of department stores and drugstores.

Learn stress management. If you check with your local recreation department or YMCA, you'll probably find they offer classes geared toward stress management techniques. Meditation, relaxation, visualization, biofeedback, yoga, and tai chi are just a few of the classes that can teach you how to let go of everyday stress.

● ●
Understanding the fight or flight response

Stress hormones prepare your body to cope with or run from whatever is causing your stress. These hormones:

- Contract your muscles, which strengthens them to protect you from injury.

- Speed up your metabolism to provide strength and energy.

- Make your heart beat faster.

- Speed up your digestive system to give your muscles extra nutrients.

- Dilate pupils to aid vision and sharpen your hearing.

- Speed breathing to provide more oxygen to your body.

- Help blood clot more quickly and constrict arteries, which lessens blood loss if you are injured.

● ●

Playing in the dirt is good for you

If you need a way to chill out at the end of the day and relieve stress, you don't have to go any farther than your own yard. Gazing at flowers and trees can relieve stress, lower blood pressure, and relax tense muscles.

A Canadian study found that people with Alzheimer's who were living in homes with gardens had fewer violent incidents. In fact, violence declined by 19 percent over two years. At homes without gardens, violent incidents increased by 680 percent.

Taking in some scenery may also help you heal faster. A University of Delaware study found that hospital patients with a view of a natural setting recovered from surgery nearly a day faster than patients who could only see a brick wall. They even needed less painkilling medicine.

Horticultural therapy is a growing field, and therapeutic gardens are sprouting up all over. According to the American Horticultural Therapy Association, nearly 300 hospitals around the country employ registered horticultural therapists. Many people with physical, emotional, and mental disabilities are benefiting from this unique therapy.

Horticultural therapy usually involves more than just looking at a garden. Tending to plants and helping them grow can be very relaxing and rewarding, and it's good exercise, too.

Hands-on way to relieve stress

If you're looking for a way to relieve your stress and anxiety, a therapeutic massage could be just what you need. Most people know first-hand how relaxing a massage can be, and scientific studies confirm it.

One study of nurses found that massage performed by a registered massage therapist reduced tension and pain and improved overall mood. Another study found that massage administered in the workplace reduced blood pressure levels.

And a study by the National Institutes of Health found that massage can relieve depression. New mothers who were stressed and depressed got a 20-minute massage twice a week. After four weeks, their depression and anxiety began to vanish, and they had lower levels of stress hormones.

Unlike many therapies, massage is usually free of side effects. However, one doctor did report in the *New England Journal of Medicine* that a patient experienced a ruptured blood vessel in her liver after having a deep-tissue massage. That doctor recommends that anyone taking blood-thinning medications or anyone with a liver tumor avoid deep-tissue massage.

Stroke

Stop a stroke before it starts

According to the American Stroke Association, someone in America has a stroke every 53 seconds. And strokes kill 160,000 people each year. Understanding strokes and how to avoid them may keep you from being added to the statistics.

When you have a stroke, the blood supply to your brain is cut off, either by a blockage of blood flow or by a blood vessel that ruptures and bleeds. When the blood supply to your brain is cut off, depriving it of oxygen, brain cells die.

A stroke that is caused by a blockage is called an ischemic stroke. Ischemic strokes can be caused by a blood clot that forms in your brain or neck (thrombosis), by a blood clot that forms elsewhere in your body and moves to your brain or neck (embolism), or by a severe narrowing of an artery that won't allow blood through (stenosis).

A stroke that is caused by bleeding into the brain or the area surrounding the brain is called a hemorrhagic stroke. These strokes are more often fatal than ischemic strokes. They are sometimes caused by a ruptured aneurysm — a weakened spot in an artery that bulges outward.

Just the thought of a stroke can be frightening, but you needn't feel helpless. There are things you can do to cut your risk.

Kick the habit. Smoking contributes to a build up of fatty substances that can block the main artery supplying blood to your brain. This type of blockage is the leading cause of strokes in the United States. If that doesn't convince you, consider these facts:

- nicotine in cigarettes raises blood pressure

- carbon monoxide in cigarettes reduces the amount of oxygen your blood carries to your brain

- smoking makes your blood thicker and more likely to clot

Kicking the habit isn't easy, but when you consider what smoking is doing to your body, it's worth the effort. Your doctor can recommend programs or medications that can make quitting easier.

Get in motion. Regular exercise can reduce your risk of stroke substantially because it helps keep your blood pressure under control. Researchers at Yale University found that men who walked over a mile a day cut their risk of stroke in half.

Drink more milk. High blood pressure often goes hand-in-hand with stroke. Since calcium helps control blood pressure, experts wondered if it would also reduce the risk of stroke. Researchers looked at information gathered for 22 years from several thousand men.

The risk of stroke was quite different among the men who took calcium pills and those who ate a lot of dairy products. Men who drank more than 16 ounces of milk a day were half as likely to suffer a stroke as those who didn't drink milk. Those who got their calcium from nondairy sources, such as supplements, had no stroke advantage.

Another study found that women who had a higher calcium intake, whether it was from food or supplements, were less likely to suffer a stroke.

These studies suggest getting plenty of calcium, particularly from dairy products, may help you avoid a stroke.

Eat cruciferous, citrus, and leafy greens. Eating at least five servings of fruits and vegetables a day may lower your stroke risk.

A recent study found that the risk of ischemic stroke was 31 percent lower in people who ate more than five servings of fruits and vegetables a day, compared with people who ate less than three servings a day. Cruciferous vegetables, like broccoli, cabbage, and cauliflower; green leafy vegetables; and citrus fruits and juices were associated with the greatest protective effect.

Buy into B vitamins. Studies have shown that B vitamins can help lower your risk of suffering a heart attack or stroke by controlling homocysteine levels. This substance, a by-product of protein metabolism, can damage and narrow your arteries.

Taking B vitamins after a stroke may even help heal the damage. In a recent study, researchers divided 50 stroke survivors into two groups. One group took a vitamin supplement containing 1 milligram (mg) of vitamin B12, 100 mg of vitamin B6, and 5 mg of folic acid. The other group took a vitamin supplement without the B vitamins. After three months, the people who were taking the vitamin supplements with the B vitamins had lower levels of homocysteine and thrombomodulin, a chemical indicator of blood vessel damage.

Another study found that even among young women, high homocysteine levels were associated with a higher risk of stroke. In the study on women ages 15 to 44, those with the highest levels of homocysteine had double the risk of stroke compared with women having lower levels.

Get plenty of potassium. If you want to lower your risk of stroke, make sure you get enough potassium in your diet. A recent study found that men who had the highest potassium intake were 38 percent less likely to have a stroke than men who had the lowest intake of potassium. Foods high in potassium include bananas, dried apricots, avocado, figs, beans, and cantaloupe.

• •
Watch out for hidden vitamin K

If you're taking warfarin or another anticoagulant, your doctor has probably told you to get a consistent amount of vitamin K in your diet. That's because vitamin K is involved in your blood's ability to clot properly. Too much or too little could interfere with your medication's effectiveness.

You may be unaware that vitamin K may have been added to snack foods made with olestra, a fat substitute. That's because olestra interferes with absorption of fat-soluble vitamins.

Although the Food and Drug Administration says the added vitamin K shouldn't have any impact on people taking anticoagulants, if you're monitoring your vitamin K intake, be aware that snacks or other foods containing olestra may contain added vitamin K.

• •

Aspirin therapy — look before you leap

Doctors often recommend daily aspirin therapy to head off heart attacks, but is it a good idea to take aspirin to ward off strokes?

Researchers have found that aspirin helps prevent recurrences in people who have already had a heart attack or stroke, but they aren't sure whether healthy people with no history of heart or artery disease should use aspirin to prevent a first heart attack or stroke.

Ischemic strokes, the most common kind, are caused by blood clots. Since aspirin helps keep blood cells slippery and less likely to clump up, it may help prevent this type of stroke. For the same reason, however, it may increase your risk of hemorrhagic stroke.

The reason may be the amount. In a recent study of almost 80,000 women, those who took one to six tablets of aspirin per week had a lower risk of ischemic stroke, but women who took more than 15 tablets per week were approximately twice as likely to suffer hemorrhagic strokes.

The risk was even higher for older women with high blood pressure. They were three times more likely to have a hemorrhagic stroke if they took more than 15 aspirin a week than women who took lower doses.

If you would like to try aspirin therapy, talk it over with your doctor first.

• •
Stroke symptoms? Call 911!

When it comes to stroke, timing is everything. A delay in treatment could mean the difference between life and death, or between complete recovery and living with paralysis.

A drug called tissue plasminogen activator or tPA (trade name: Activase) dissolves blood clots that cause ischemic strokes, making recovery more likely. For tPA to be effective, it must be given within three hours of the stroke.

It's important to know the warning signs of stroke:

• Numbness or weakness of an arm or leg, especially on one side of the body

• Sudden confusion or trouble speaking

• Dizziness

• Loss of balance or coordination

• Blurred or double vision

• Sudden, severe unexplained headache

If you think you are having a stroke, call for emergency medical help immediately.

• •

TMJ

Put the bite on TMJ

Do you have unexplained headaches and problems with your jaw, like pain when yawning, funny noises when you move it, or difficulty moving it from side to side. If so, you may have temporomandibular joint syndrome (TMJ).

TMJ is a disorder that affects the joint connecting your lower jaw to your head. This "hinge" is very complicated and quite unstable, even though the muscles that work the jaw are among the most powerful in your body. When you think of the tremendous pressure you use when biting and chewing, and the range of motion your jaw is capable of, it is no surprise that the joint can be easily damaged.

A big step in successful treatment of TMJ is an accurate diagnosis. It is often misdiagnosed as migraines, sinus infections, or other dental problems. Once you have identified the source of your pain, you can start relieving it.

Unclench. Clenching your jaw is a habit. You may do it a thousand times a day and not even be aware of it. Everyone reacts to stress differently, but if you find that you clench your jaw when you are tense, angry, or upset, try channeling that energy into something not so destructive, like squeezing a soft rubber ball or whistling.

Stop grinding your teeth. This is another habit you may not even know you have, but if your spouse says you grind your teeth in your sleep, see your dentist. She can fit you with a nighttime mouthpiece that will force your jaws apart.

Ice it down — heat it up. Cold compresses followed by moist heat can ease the spasms in your jaw muscles.

Rub it out. Massaging the muscles in your neck, back, shoulders, and face can soothe the soreness and relax the tension. After you've warmed up your face with compresses and massage, stretch your jaw muscles, but do it gently. You want to relieve the muscle spasms that accompany TMJ, not cause further injury.

Toss that pillow and turn over. The way you sleep at night can affect how you feel the next day. Using pillows and sleeping on your stomach puts an unnatural strain on your neck. Instead, roll up a soft towel, place it under your neck, and then sleep on your back.

Chew softly. Hard, chewy foods will make your jaw work harder. Try eating mostly soft foods and avoid chewing gum.

Stop the swelling. Over-the-counter pain relievers, like ibuprofen, will not only make you more comfortable, they will ease the inflammation in your damaged jaw muscles.

Listen to your body. Certain foods and drugs can increase the tension in some people by speeding up their metabolisms. Caffeine and decongestants are two examples. If coffee tends to make you jittery, you could end up unconsciously clenching your jaw even more, so cut back or switch to decaf. If your cold medicine is making you jumpy, try another product.

Dial your dentist. If the shape of your jaw or the alignment of your teeth is the cause of your TMJ, you may have no choice but to seek professional help. Your dentist can fit you with a custom mouthguard that will take the pressure off your jaw muscles and allow the spasms to relax, or he might recommend orthodontics to move your teeth into their proper position. He can also grind the surfaces of your teeth to allow them to match up more evenly. If all else fails, he might recommend orthopedic surgery to shift your jaw bone. Don't rush into these last procedures. Think over all your options and get a second opinion.

• •

Proper posture improves TMJ

Texas researchers have found a new way to treat your TMJ symptoms — improve your posture.

Researchers divided people with TMJ into two groups. Both groups were given self-management instructions, but one group also received training for proper head and neck posture from physical therapists.

The people who received posture training averaged a 42-percent decrease in TMJ symptoms, while the ones who only received self-management instructions had an average 8-percent reduction in symptoms.

Maybe your mother was right when she nagged you about your posture. It's important in more ways than you know.

• •

Ulcers

6 ways to beat an ulcer

"Calm down, you're going to give yourself an ulcer." Have you ever heard those words? Historically, people who didn't handle stress well seemed to be more likely to get ulcers. Although stress and lifestyle can make them worse, most ulcers are caused by tiny, spiral-shaped bacteria called *Helicobacter pylori*.

These bacteria penetrate your stomach's protective lining, making it more susceptible to damage from digestive acids. They also cause your stomach to produce too much acid, contributing even more to the development of a painful ulcer.

Your doctor can do a simple blood test to see if you are infected with this bacteria. If you are, he'll probably prescribe antibiotics to kill the bacteria. He might also recommend the following lifestyle changes.

Stop smoking. Cigarette smoking increases your risk of developing an ulcer. It also makes existing ulcers heal more slowly and increases the likelihood that your ulcers will return after they've finally healed.

Limit stress. Although stress is no longer considered the major cause of ulcers, many people with ulcers say emotional stress increases the pain. Physical stress, such as surgery or a serious injury, may trigger the formation of ulcers.

Don't overdo NSAIDs. Nonsteroidal anti-inflammatory drugs (NSAIDs) can undermine your stomach's natural protection. Aspirin and ibuprofen are common NSAIDs taken for arthritis, headaches, and minor aches and pains. If they are causing you stomach pain, ask your doctor about switching to another type of pain reliever.

Fill up on fiber. A recent study by Harvard University researchers states that eating lots of high-fiber fruits and vegetables means a lower risk of developing ulcers. Your digestive system will get the most benefit from insoluble fibers, the tough, indigestible parts of certain foods that will not dissolve in water. Foods high in this kind of fiber are wheat bran, whole wheat breads, brown rice, beans, fruits, and vegetables.

Eat colorful fruits and veggies. This same study gave vitamin A high marks for preventing ulcers. The next time you're food shopping choose the most colorful fruits and vegetables you can find. These are the richest sources of beta carotene, which turns into vitamin A in your body. Whether you choose apricots, sweet potatoes, carrots or spinach, or take supplements or multivitamins, you'll be protecting your body from the pain of stomach ulcers.

Avoid certain beverages. Alcohol, black tea, and coffee, even decaffeinated, are all known to irritate your digestive tract. While drinking these products may not give you an ulcer, they can make the one you have feel worse — and maybe even take longer to heal. It may be hard to give up your morning cup of java, but try substituting a hot drink that is milder on your stomach. Chinese green tea is an excellent choice. In fact, it's a potent antioxidant that can also protect you from heart disease and cancer.

• •
The lowdown on milk

Years ago, many people believed drinking milk eased the pain of ulcers. They thought dairy foods soothed and coated the stomach lining, protecting the inflamed tissue and giving it a chance to heal.

During this time, medical evidence indicated that milk might actually slow down the healing process of ulcers. Researchers said milk proteins cause the stomach to produce gastric acid, which could irritate the ulcers more.

But a recent study found that milk may protect your stomach because it makes it difficult for *Helicobacter pylori*, the bacterium responsible for some ulcers, to get a grip on your stomach lining.

While drinking milk may not help an existing ulcer heal, it might keep you from getting one in the first place.

● ●

Possible new ulcer treatment causes buzz

Bees are busy and useful creatures indeed. They have supplied us with honey for food and medicine for centuries, and new research shows that another bee product may help us heal ulcers as well.

Propolis, a material bees use in making and maintaining their hives, has long been used as a home remedy and has a reputation as an antibacterial.

Researchers tested propolis solutions of varying strength against 20 different strains of ulcer-causing *H. pylori* bacteria in the laboratory. A solution containing no propolis had no effect on *H. pylori,* but many of the propolis solutions slowed the growth of the bacteria.

The next step is to test propolis in humans. If it works, our busy little friends may soon give us an effective way to treat ulcers and other bacterial infections.

Urinary disorders

Natural ways to sidestep painful infections

The pain and burning of a urinary tract infection (UTI) can make the bathroom your least favorite place to be.

Women are more likely to develop UTIs than men, although men over 50 often get them because of an enlarged prostate. Anything that interferes with urine flow can contribute to an infection. The longer urine stays in your urinary tract, the more time bacteria have to get a grip and multiply.

If you think you have a UTI, see your doctor. Ask him to take a urine sample to be sure you really have a UTI before he prescribes antibiotics. Many antibiotics have unpleasant side effects, including kidney damage.

These natural strategies may help heal a UTI or prevent you from getting one in the future.

Stock up on cranberry juice. This tart juice may be a delicious way to keep UTIs from cramping your style. Some doctors think cranberries slow the growth of bacteria by making your urine more acidic. Other studies show that cranberries keep bacteria from clinging to your urinary tract. The bacteria just slip right through and out of your body.

However it works, to prevent UTIs, you may want to add about 3 ounces of cranberry juice to your diet every day. One study found that the protective effects of cranberry juice appeared only after four to eight weeks. For the most protection, drink cranberry juice regularly.

Wash it away with water. Most doctors agree that water can help wash bacteria out of your body. Drink at least six to eight glasses of water every day. If your urine is pale yellow, you're getting enough. A dark color means you need to visit the water fountain a little more often.

Take some vitamin C. Like cranberry juice, vitamin C supplements may make your urine more acidic, thus making it more difficult for bacteria to grow.

Help yourself to herbs. Some herbs, like goldenrod and parsley, can increase your urine flow, making you less likely to get a UTI. You can find them at your local health food store, or look for fresh parsley in your grocery store.

The next time you find some decorative parsley on your plate, don't just toss it aside. Try eating it for an extra bit of urinary protection. But beware of staying outdoors too long afterward. Parsley can increase your sensitivity to the sun.

Another herb, bearberry, has an antiseptic effect so it neutralizes bacteria before it can do its dirty work. Bearberry was used effectively for years to battle UTIs before sulfa drugs and antibiotics came along. Unfortunately, this herb can be toxic. If you have kidney disease, consult your doctor before trying any herb for UTIs.

Don't fight the urge. Go to the bathroom whenever you feel the need, and empty your bladder completely each time. You may be tempted to resist the urge to urinate if you're too busy to bother, or you think it's going to be painful. Just remember — the longer urine sits in your bladder, the more likely it is to stagnate and allow bacteria to grow.

Be careful how you wipe. If you're a woman, don't wipe from back to front. You may drag bacteria from your anus toward your urethra, giving germs a chance to set off an infection.

Urinate before and after sex. Emptying your bladder before and after sexual intercourse washes bacteria out of your urethra.

Keep it clean. Keep the area around the urethral opening as clean as possible. Make sure your genital area and your partner's are clean before intercourse to reduce the risk of a bacterial infection.

Ditch the diaphragm. If you use a diaphragm for birth control, try another method. Diaphragms press against the bladder and prevent it from emptying completely. This increases your likelihood of infection. Also, most women leave the diaphragm in for eight to 10 hours. This time span allows bacteria to multiply and cause infection.

Take a shower instead of a bath. Baths may be relaxing but sitting in a tub of water may give bacteria an opportunity to enter your urethra. Take showers instead.

Skip the douches and sprays. If your skin is sensitive, keep powders, soaps, creams, bath oils and gels, and other hygiene products away from your genital area. Scented douches and feminine hygiene sprays may smell pretty, but they can also irritate your urethra.

Stop smoking. In case you need another reason to ditch your cigarettes, smoking increases your risk for bladder infections.

Ask about new treatments. If you are postmenopausal, talk with your doctor about using a vaginal estrogen cream. It may help reduce the risk of UTIs.

And be on the lookout for a vaccine against this common infection. Although still experimental, researchers hope it will prevent *E. coli* bacteria from attaching to the sides of your urinary tract and causing an infection.

Take extra precautions. Although a recent study discounted many of the old recommendations for preventing UTIs, if you're prone to these infections, taking extra precautions can't hurt. Try wearing cotton panties instead of nylon, avoiding tight pants, wearing thigh-high stockings rather than pantyhose, and avoiding tampons or changing them often if you do use them.

If you end up with a bladder infection despite your best efforts, take care of it right away. That means seeing your doctor. Putting off treatment could allow the bacteria to travel to your kidneys or into your bloodstream, causing a more serious infection. Frequent, painful urination, as well as fever, lower back pain, chills, nausea, and confusion, are symptoms of a kidney infection. An untreated kidney infection can cause permanent kidney damage.

Help for a leaky bladder

Over 200 million people have bladder control problems, and many of them find the situation so embarrassing they won't even mention it to their doctors. Women are more often affected than men, and the chances that you'll experience it increase with age.

If you're having problems controlling your bladder, tell your doctor. There are effective treatments available for urinary incontinence. In the meantime, here are some ways you can help yourself.

Check your menu. Many foods and drinks affect your ability to hold urine. Watch your intake of coffee, tea, carbonated drinks, citrus fruits, tomatoes, chocolate, sugar, honey, spicy foods, and milk products. Perhaps one or more of these are adding to your problem.

Drink lots of water. Don't try to control your incontinence by drinking less. It is still important to keep your body well-hydrated. Experts recommend six to eight glasses of water each day.

Take care of your skin. If your incontinence continues, the skin that comes in contact with urine may become irritated and infected. Keep your skin clean and dry by using mild soap, warm water, and soft towels. Ask your pharmacist to recommend a cream or ointment to help protect your skin.

Don't be ashamed to wear pads. You can wear an absorbent product to give you peace of mind and let you participate in activities you enjoy.

Train your bladder. By going to the bathroom on a strict schedule, you teach your bladder to hold more urine. Keep a chart or diary and begin by going to the toilet every 30 minutes. Gradually increase the time to every two to three hours.

Buy into biofeedback. A professional can train you in this technique to help you become more aware of how your body works. This will help you gain more control over your bladder.

Stay active. Exercising regularly will contribute to your over-all health and keep your bowel movements regular. Constipation can affect incontinence.

Stop smoking. Tobacco smoke affects your bladder and ure-thra. And that hacking smoker's cough places a lot of stress on your bladder, which can lead to leakage. It's never too late to quit. Ask your doctor for help.

Work out. Kegel exercises are a great way to strengthen the muscles that control your urine flow. Sit comfortably with your legs uncrossed and your abdominal, thigh, and buttocks muscles relaxed. Then pretend you are trying to stop urinating. Keep these muscles tense for about 10 seconds, then relax. Repeat this tensing and relaxing 10 times, three times a day. Be patient. You may not see any improvement for at least six to eight weeks, and you may have to make the exercises part of your daily routine.

If you want to be sure you are doing them right, you can buy vaginal cones. Insert one of the weighted plastic cones into your vagina and tighten the muscles to hold the cone in place. If you are doing the Kegels correctly, the cone will not fall out. Remember to tighten these muscles before you cough, sneeze, or lift a heavy object to help control any leaking. Soon, you may not even have to think about it.

•
Could hair dyes cause bladder cancer?

Maybe, says new research that suggests the search for the perfect hair color could increase your risk for cancer of the bladder.

The study found that women who dyed their hair once a month or more for 15 years or longer were three times as likely to develop bladder cancer as those who didn't dye their hair or dyed it less often. Hairdressers or barbers were five times as likely to get the disease.

More research is needed to confirm the findings, and study results only included women who used permanent hair dyes. However, if you dye your hair often, you might want to consider using a semi-permanent dye.

• •

Weight gain

The only 'diet' you'll ever need

After all the trendy diets you've tried, aren't you ready for an ultimate, sensible eating plan — one designed to help you maintain a healthy weight and prevent disease?

Several major health organizations — American Heart Association, American Cancer Society, American Dietetic Association, American Academy of Pediatrics, and National Institutes of Health — joined forces to develop the Unified Dietary Guidelines.

These guidelines were designed to prevent disease by helping control obesity and encouraging you to eat a variety of healthy foods. Here are some of the recommendations:

- **Fat.** No more than 30 percent of total calories from all types of fat, including 10 percent or less from saturated fat.

- **Carbohydrates.** Complex carbohydrates, such as cereals, grains, fruits, and vegetables, should make up 55 percent or more of your total daily calories.

- **Cholesterol.** You should limit dietary cholesterol to 300 milligrams a day or less.

- **Salt.** You shouldn't eat more than 6 grams (one teaspoon) of salt a day.

- **Calories.** Don't consume more calories than you need to maintain a desirable body weight.

Everyone needs a different number of calories to maintain weight or lose weight. A doctor could help you determine your specific needs, but here are some examples:

If a 55-year-old woman who is 5'5" tall and weighs 135 pounds does four hours of very light activity, like reading or driving, and 30 minutes of light activity, like sweeping or walking, she would need 1,705 calories a day to maintain her current weight.

If a 55-year-old man who is 5'10" tall and weighs 155 pounds does four hours of very light activity and 30 minutes of light activity, he would need 1,975 calories to maintain his current weight.

The guidelines don't tell you exactly what to eat and how much, like most eating plans. Instead, you use your own judgment to stay within the guidelines. The best way to do this is to eat a variety of foods, especially foods from plant sources, like grains, fruits, and vegetables.

If you have any health problems, talk with your doctor before changing your diet.

●●●●●●●●●●●●●●●●●●●●●●●●●●●

What's your BMI?

Being overweight isn't just a matter of appearance — it can push you into an early grave. According to a recent study of over a million people, being overweight significantly increases your risk of early death from all causes, including heart disease and cancer.

If you struggle to keep the weight off, you're not alone. About half of Americans are considered overweight, and one out of every five adults in the United States is clinically obese.

Body mass index (BMI) is the best way to judge whether you are at a healthy weight. For women, a BMI between 19.1 to 25.8 is considered healthy, while a BMI greater than 25.8 to 27.3 is considered slightly overweight with some health risks. The higher a woman's BMI goes above 27.3, the greater the health risks.

Because men generally have more muscle mass than women, their average BMIs are slightly higher. Men with a BMI of 20.7 to 26.4 are considered healthy. A BMI greater than 26.4 to 27.8 is considered slightly overweight with some health risks. These risks increase significantly for men with BMIs over 31.1.

Use this chart to determine your BMI.

Body mass index (BMI) chart

Weight	100	110	120	130	140	150	160	170	180	190	200
Height											
5'0"	20	21	23	25	27	29	31	33	35	37	39
5'1"	19	21	23	25	26	28	30	32	34	36	38
5'2"	18	20	22	24	26	27	29	31	33	35	37
5'3"	18	19	21	23	25	27	28	30	32	34	35
5'4"	17	19	21	22	24	26	27	29	31	33	34
5'5"	17	18	20	22	23	25	27	28	30	32	33
5'6"	16	18	19	21	23	24	26	27	29	31	32
5'7"	16	17	19	20	22	23	25	27	28	30	31
5'8"	15	17	18	20	21	23	24	26	27	29	30
5'9"	15	16	18	19	21	22	24	25	27	28	30
5'10"	14	16	17	19	20	22	23	24	26	27	29
5'11"	14	15	17	18	20	21	22	24	25	26	28
6'0"	14	15	16	18	19	20	22	23	24	26	27
6'1"	13	15	16	17	18	20	21	22	24	25	26
6'2"	13	14	15	17	18	19	21	22	23	24	26
6'3"	12	14	15	16	17	19	20	21	22	24	25

• • • • • • • • • • • • • • • • • • • •

How to tame your cravings

If you're trying to peel off a few pounds, giving into cravings can really wreck your weight loss plan. Here are some tips to help.

Feast on fiber. It's easy to give in to cravings when your stomach is growling, so eat foods that are satisfying and filling — foods full of fiber, protein, and water. Researchers have found boiled potatoes to be especially satisfying. Beans and lentils, because of their high-fiber content and your body's tendency to absorb them slowly, also make you feel full longer.

Munch on mini-meals. Eating five or six small meals, instead of three big ones, helps stabilize your blood sugar levels. This will keep you from getting so hungry you end up stuffing yourself at the next meal. If you're watching your weight, divide your daily calories among the five or six meals. Just because you're eating more meals doesn't mean you need to eat more calories. You simply need to spread them out better.

Don't crash diet. Most crash diets are destined for failure — quick weight loss is rarely permanent weight loss. Depriving yourself severely can lead to an increase in cravings because nerve chemicals and hormones go wildly out of whack on quick weight loss diets.

Snack wisely. If you're craving crunchy, opt for pretzels instead of potato chips. Even better, crunch on carrots or an apple. To calm a raging chocolate craving, try some sugar-free cocoa. If you're cruising for something creamy, try hot cereals, like oatmeal, or reduced fat and sugar soups and puddings.

● ●
Here's good news for chocoholics

Sometimes you just *have* to have chocolate — especially if you're a woman. Researchers have found that 40 percent of women and 15 percent of men experience chocolate cravings. And those cravings are real, according to a recent report.

It's debatable exactly what causes that craving, but researchers believe it is probably a combination of factors.

Chocolate naturally contains certain compounds also found in the brain. These compounds help regulate mood. A little chocolate pick-me-up when you're down may actually be a form of self-medication. Chocolate cravings seem to hit women just before menstruation, when hormone levels may trigger cravings for fatty foods — and chocolate is full of fat, as well as sugar. Many people believe they crave chocolate just because it tastes so good.

Chocolate's taste, chemical properties, and nutrients, like magnesium, may provide just the right combination to form one of the world's most craved foods. But don't use that as an excuse to eat candy bars every day. Too much fat and sugar causes too much fat on your body. If you eat a balanced diet, you can indulge your "chocolate tooth" in small amounts and feel no guilt. You really do need that chocolate bar.

• •

Don't get burned by 'miracle' diets

Visit any bookstore and you'll see shelves in the health section crammed with diet books. Are these diets healthy, or would they be more appropriately shelved in the fiction section?

Although you'll probably lose weight if you follow one of these diets, most of them are designed for short-term weight loss. As soon as you go off the diet, you'll gain the weight back. Worse than that, some of them may damage your health by promoting poor eating habits.

The American Dietetic Association recently warned against high-protein, high-fat, low-carbohydrate diets. These diets are very popular because of books like *Dr. Atkins' Diet Revolution, Mastering the Zone,* and *The Carbohydrate Addict's Diet.*

High-protein diets promote short-term weight loss through a process called ketosis. Ketosis occurs whenever you're not getting enough carbohydrates to fuel your body. Carbohydrates are normally one of your body's main sources of energy. During ketosis, your body turns to other energy sources, including protein. When protein is used for energy, you lose weight because the protein isn't available for its usual job — to build and replace tissue.

Most people can't stick with one of these diets for long. That's probably a good thing because some of them contain more fat and cholesterol than health experts recommend. They may also be low in fruits and vegetables. Numerous studies have found that fruits and vegetables protect against many life-threatening diseases, including cancer.

A recent study found that high levels of protein over time can raise homocysteine levels in your blood, contributing to heart and artery disease. A long-term, high-protein diet may also stress your kidneys and liver.

Despite the complicated weight loss plans advocated in many popular books, the best way to lose weight is simple — eat less and exercise more, and it's still the only way to keep weight off.

Little changes add up to big weight loss

Little changes in lifestyle can add up to big changes in weight. That should be encouraging news to anyone struggling with weight loss. Every time you pass up dessert, every time you park a little farther from the store, you're adding fuel to your personal weight-loss fire. Here are a few more examples of small but helpful changes anyone can make.

Chew gum. A recent study found that chewing gum increases the number of calories you burn by 20 percent. People in the study burned an average of 11 more calories an hour while chewing gum than they did when they were not chewing gum.

Eleven calories may not sound like a lot, but if you chewed gum during your waking hours and made no other dietary or lifestyle changes, you would lose about 10 pounds in a year. Even if you don't choose to chew all day long, this study shows how little changes really can add up to big weight loss.

Fidget. Your mom probably taught you not to fidget. But new studies suggest that people who fidget burn more calories than people who don't. Researchers call this "fidget factor" NEAT (nonexercise activity thermogenesis), and say it accounts for an average of 348 calories burned a day.

Tapping your toes or drumming your fingers may be annoying to the people around you, but if you do it when you're alone, you could burn off some pounds with very little effort.

Eat in. If you limit how often you eat out, you may save money and lose weight. A recent study found that the more often people ate in restaurants, the more overweight they were likely to be. Researchers theorize that the increase in restaurant eating in the United States could be responsible in part for the national rise in obesity statistics.

Keep it small. According to a recent survey by the American Institute for Cancer Research, people in the United States believe that, when it comes to weight control, the kind of food they eat is more important than how much. The survey also found that people underestimate portion size. Although the kind of food you eat is important, eating too much of any food — even low-fat foods — adds unnecessary calories and weight.

One way to keep your portions under control is to buy smaller containers of food. A recent study by a University of Chicago at Urbana-Champaign researcher found that when people ate popcorn from a large container, they consumed 44 percent more than people who were eating from smaller containers. If you buy food in small containers rather than the jumbo economy size, you may eat less.

While you're working on smaller portions, some people find that it helps to use smaller plates. It takes less to fill the plate up, and you're less likely to go back for seconds than to clean your first plate.

Each of these small changes may not make a huge and immediate difference in your weight. But if you make several small changes and give it time, you may be pleasantly surprised by the difference you'll see.

● ●
Easy way to curb your appetite

Looking for an easy way to trick yourself into consuming fewer calories? If so, you've probably tried drinking large glasses of ice water before meals to curb your out-of-control appetite.

Drinking water is a good idea, but it may not be an effective appetite suppressant. A recent study, however, found that if you eat foods with a high water content, you'll consume fewer calories.

Researchers gave women either a chicken-rice casserole, the same casserole with a glass of water, or the casserole with a bowl of chicken-rice soup. Although the meals contained the same ingredients in the same amounts, when the women ate the soup with the casserole, their appetites were satisfied sooner.

Researchers say that soup isn't the only food that has this effect. Any food high in water, like fruits, vegetables, and pasta with vegetables, may help you satisfy your appetite with fewer calories.

● ●

Surprising reasons to exercise every day

To lose weight, you must burn more calories than you take in — but weight loss programs without exercise are doomed to failure.

In one study, researchers compared the lifestyles, weight, and body fat of 485 pairs of female twins. They found that the women who exercised most frequently were more likely to have low body fat. Even the women who had an overweight twin were less likely to be obese if they exercised regularly. This suggests that exercise fights weight gain even in people who have a hereditary predisposition to obesity.

If you don't exercise to lose weight, exercise for your health. You're more likely to live a longer, healthier life if you stay active. Here are just some of the ways exercise helps keep you healthy.

Cuts cancer risk. Exercise may be a good defense against breast, uterine, and colon cancers. Here's why:

- Reduces fat. Colon cancer risk, which seems to be boosted by too much weight, is lowered by exercise. A weekly game of tennis or a couple of hours of brisk walking can lower your risk of developing colon cancer by 30 percent, according to Harvard researchers. And those who exercised even more — running more than four hours a week or walking more than 12 — cut their risk by more than 50 percent.

- Boosts your immune system. Exercise stimulates macrophages, a type of white blood cell in your immune system. These cells are your first line of defense against invaders, like viruses and bacteria. Because exercise slightly damages soft tissue, macrophages are routinely called upon to make repairs. This may keep them in shape for fighting tumor cells.

- Lowers the amount of estrogen in a woman's body — a culprit in breast and uterine cancers. One recent study suggests that moderate, regular physical activity can cut a woman's risk of developing breast cancer by as much as 60 percent. The greatest benefit came from exercising four hours a week, but even two or three hours of exercise weekly appears to help.

- Lowers your insulin levels. Inactive people may be more likely to develop colon cancer because they have higher insulin levels than exercisers. Insulin, a hormone your body uses to help metabolize sugar, encourages tumors to grow in animals and perhaps in humans. Exercise reduces the amount of insulin your body needs because it makes you more sensitive to the hormone.

Helps defeat diabetes. People who have diabetes, either insulin-dependent or noninsulin-dependent, will benefit from exercise because physical activity helps the body use insulin more efficiently. In fact, one study found that just 40 minutes a week of moderate exercise can reduce your risk of developing type II diabetes by 50 percent. Recommended exercises include brisk walking, slow swimming, light bicycling, easy aerobic dance, tennis, basketball, and using a treadmill or stepping machine. Because diabetes frequently causes eye and foot problems, ask your doctor's advice about setting up an exercise program if you are diabetic.

Keeps bones strong. It's exercise, not just milk, that builds strong bones. Researchers from Tufts University's Center on Aging found that doing 45 minutes of weight-lifting exercises twice a week improves strength, bone density, and balance. The result? Fewer falls and fewer fractures. Researchers say bones are like muscle — if you don't use them, you lose them.

Boosts your brain power. You know it's smart to exercise, but did you know people who exercise are smarter? Research shows physical exercise can encourage creativity, speed your thinking, and even help you beat the blues. By flooding the brain with more blood, aerobic exercise fuels brain cells with oxygen and nutrients. That may be why exercise can boost your reaction time and improve the speed at which you process information. It can even improve your mood. According to researchers, 30 to 60 minutes of aerobic exercise increases the amount of a mood-lifting brain chemical called serotonin. One study found that aerobic exercise is just as effective as psychotherapy in helping mild depression.

Strengthens your heart. You can cut your heart attack risk in half just by walking 30 to 45 minutes three times a week. Without exercise, your heart gradually loses its ability to circulate blood. People who have already had heart attacks also benefit from exercise as long as they have their doctor's OK. In one study, men with chronic heart failure improved blood flow just by exercising their forearms.

If you already have heart disease, be careful not to overdo it when you start an exercise program. Vigorous exercise, like snow shoveling, can cause heart attacks in people with heart disease who are usually inactive; smoke; or have high blood pressure, high cholesterol, or diabetes.

Stops a stroke before it starts. You don't need to run a marathon to reduce your risk of stroke. Walking just three blocks a day lowered risk 30 percent and walking a mile, about five blocks, cut risk in half for men between the ages of 50 and 60 in a recent study. This seems to be true even if you smoke or have high blood pressure or diabetes, say researchers. Imagine the benefits if you don't have these other risk factors.

Help for exercise-related skin injuries

You're exercising regularly and feeling great, but now you have an embarrassing skin injury. These common ailments are treatable and preventable.

Runner's rump. Joggers and long-distance runners may experience redness, soreness, and sometimes swelling between the buttocks, on the upper thighs, or in the groin area. Runner's rump will go away in a day or two if you cut back on running. You can also try wearing silky nylon running shorts or Lycra leggings because these fabrics aren't as likely to rub and aggravate the problem.

Jogger's nipple. This condition most often occurs in long-distance runners. It is caused by coarse fabric rubbing against the nipples for long periods of time. Use lotion on the affected area and wear shirts made of soft, silky fabrics. Women should make sure their bras fit properly to avoid shifting and moving while they are running.

Surfer's nodule. These are small bumps that appear on your kneecaps, shins, or ankles where your skin comes in contact with the surfboard. Stay away from your surfboard for a while to let them heal.

Black palm. Golfers, tennis players, and weightlifters all have this problem occasionally. It looks like the palm of your hand is bruised. This is caused by sudden choppy movements that tear the delicate blood vessels in your palm. It goes away in time, but to avoid this problem in the future, wear athletic gloves.

Tennis toe. This painful ailment is the bruising and discoloration of your big toe due to repeated and sudden starts and stops that jam the big toe into the front of the shoe. Joggers, racquetball players, and skiers may also have this problem. To avoid tennis toe, keep your toenails trimmed and make sure your shoes fit properly.

Weight loss wonders or dangerous drugs?

While obesity can't be treated with medication for the rest of your life, sometimes you need a little extra help to get you started down the weight loss road. Here's a guide to some of the products available.

Prescription drugs. Your doctor can prescribe drugs designed to help you lose weight. Unfortunately, many of these drugs have serious side effects and should only be used by people who are so overweight the dangers of the excess weight are greater than the potential side effects of the drugs. They aren't appropriate for someone who just wants to lose 10 pounds before a high school reunion.

- **Appetite suppressants.** Most prescription weight loss drugs work by suppressing your appetite. Two of these drugs, fenfluramine and dexfenfluramine, were taken off the market because they were associated with serious heart problems. Prescription appetite suppressants still available include phentermine (brand names: Adipex-P, Fastin, Ionamin, Oby-trim), sibutramine (brand name: Meridia), diethylpropion (brand name: Tenuate), mazindol (brand names: Sanorex, Mazanor), and phendimetrazine (brand names: Bontril, Plegine, Prelu-2, X-Trozine). People who take these medications generally lose an average of 5 to 22 pounds more than they would with nondrug obesity treatments. You shouldn't take them long-term because their safety and effectiveness beyond one year hasn't been established.

- **Orlistat.** The newest diet drug on the market, Orlistat (brand name: Xenical), doesn't work by suppressing appetite. Instead, it blocks fat absorption by about 30 percent. According to a two-year study, orlistat was effective in helping people lose weight and keep it off. It also improved cholesterol and insulin levels. A word of caution — because it inhibits fat absorption, it may interfere with your ability to absorb fat-soluble vitamins A, D, E, and K. Ask your doctor about taking supplements. Side effects may include intestinal cramping, gas, and rectal leakage.

Over-the-counter supplements. You can buy many products at the drugstore that claim to help you lose weight. Some of them may help, but any weight loss you might experience is usually gained back as soon as you stop taking the product. You have to make permanent changes in the way you eat to achieve permanent changes in your weight and health. If you decide to try supplements, do your homework and know what you're taking and what side effects you can expect. Here are a few examples.

- **Pyruvate.** One nutritional supplement, pyruvate, may be effective in helping you lose weight. In one recent study, researchers divided 26 people into two groups. One group took pyruvate, and the other group took a placebo. Both groups exercised three days a week. After six weeks, the pyruvate group lost a significant amount of weight and body fat and had more energy. The placebo group also had more energy, but they didn't lose weight or body fat. Researchers say pyruvate may work to promote weight loss by raising metabolism while lowering insulin levels. Pyruvate is found in small amounts in red apples, cheese, dark beer, and red wine.

- **Fiber supplements.** Fiber supplements, like Metamucil, may help promote weight loss. Supplements containing psyllium may be particularly effective. A small study found that women who took plantago seed granules, from which psyllium is made, before a meal felt significantly fuller one hour after the meal than women who had taken a placebo. In addition, the women who used psyllium ate less fat. Other studies have found that psyllium helps improve cholesterol levels. If you decide to take fiber supplements, start with small amounts and gradually increase. A sudden increase in fiber intake could cause abdominal discomfort. Don't forget you can always increase your fiber intake naturally by eating more fiber-rich foods, like whole grains and fruits and vegetables.

- **Appetite suppressants.** Most over-the-counter diet aids, like Dexatrim and Acutrim, contain phenylpropanolamine (PPA). This drug is used as a nasal decongestant, but it also works as an appetite suppressant. It clears nasal congestion by narrowing blood vessels, which could also raise blood pressure in people with high blood pressure. You should limit your intake of caffeine when taking any product that contains PPA. Like prescription appetite suppressants, they aren't meant to be taken long-term.

- **Ephedra.** Many people may be unaware that some weight loss supplements, such as Metabolife 356 and Meta-lite, contain ephedra, often in combination with caffeine. Ephedra is an herbal stimulant that has been implicated in 35 deaths. It is also known as ma huang and is found in herbal supplements like Herbal Ecstacy and Herbal Phen-Fen. Side effects of ephedra include an increase in blood pressure, heartbeat irregularities, insomnia, seizures, heart attack, and stroke. The Food and Drug Administration (FDA) has proposed limiting the amount of ephedrine, the active chemical in ephedra, manufacturers are allowed to put in their products. If you take products containing ephedra, you may want to follow recommendations in the FDA proposal — don't take more than 8 milligrams (mg) of ephedrine alkaloids in a six-hour period or more than 24 mg a day. The FDA also recommends that you don't use the product for more than seven days or take it with substances that have a known stimulant effect, like caffeine or yohimbine.

Wounds and injuries

Natural ways to heal a wound and fight infection

From the first time you fell and scraped your knee as a child, you've had to deal with minor cuts, sores, and wounds. But for many people, especially those who are bedridden, sores are a serious problem. It's good to know there are natural ways to prevent infection and help these wounds heal faster.

Try honey. Almost all ancient civilizations used honey as a treatment for wounds, sores, and skin ulcers, and numerous medical studies have supported its healing power. In one recent study, people with wound infections following surgery were treated with honey or antiseptics applied to the skin. The people treated with honey healed much faster, were less likely to require re-suturing, and had less scarring than the people treated with antiseptics.

Consider super-healing sugar. Another sweetener that has been used to treat wounds is sugar. In one study, hospital workers mixed sugar with hydrogen peroxide to form a paste to put on sores, especially bedsores. The study found that the paste worked well if used early in the healing process. But, if used in the later stages, the sugar acted like sandpaper and caused unnecessary bleeding.

Lower stress. If you learn stress management techniques, you could help yourself heal faster. Wounds heal more slowly on people who are under stress. Research indicates this might be because stress increases the level of certain hormones in the blood, which could slow down the healing process.

Avoid aloe. The aloe vera plant can soothe and help heal burns, but it could increase healing time for wounds. In one study, surgeons used aloe vera or standard treatment on surgical incisions. The incisions with standard treatment healed in 40 days, but the ones treated with aloe vera took 84 days to heal.

● ●

Do you need emergency medical care?

Don't hesitate to get help ...

- if your cut is still bleeding after five minutes of steady pressure.

- if you have a puncture wound caused by a nail or a bite. Dog and cat bites can be serious, but a bite from a person is more dangerous.

- if your wound has anything embedded inside, such as dirt or glass.

- if you have a cut that causes fever or swelling, or if you have numbness or trouble moving the affected area.

If you have a cut you can treat yourself, clean it under running water. The aerated sprayer on your sink is ideal for cleaning cuts and scrapes. To prevent infection, make sure you clean the cut thoroughly. Be aware that cat scratches may be especially important to clean, since they can lead to cat scratch fever.

When the cut is clean, dry it by patting with a clean, dry cloth or sterile gauze. Apply antiseptic ointment or a natural alternative and wrap with gauze.

● ●

Extraordinary results from high-tech bandage

Soldiers wounded in battle aren't the only ones who will benefit from a new blood-clotting bandage. About 50,000 people a year bleed to death from car wrecks and other trauma.

The U.S. Army Medical Command and the American Red Cross are working together to develop the bandage, which is made from clotting compounds found in human plasma.

The idea behind the bandage is to create fibrin, a sticky blood component that helps form scabs. Fibrin is formed when another substance, fibrinogen, is activated by an enzyme called thrombin at the site of a wound. Making fibrin ahead of time doesn't work because it will only stick to a wound as it is activated.

Researchers have found that they can freeze-dry fibrinogen and thrombin, and then combine them. That way, they don't turn into fibrin until they touch water or blood. The freeze-dried components are put on a dissolvable backing that can be pressed onto a wound, where the blood activates the compounds. They stop the bleeding and form an instant scab.

No one knows how much the bandages will cost when they hit the market, but if they're made from donated human blood, the cost is expected to be very high, as much as $1,000 per bandage. It may be yet another good reason to give blood.

Index